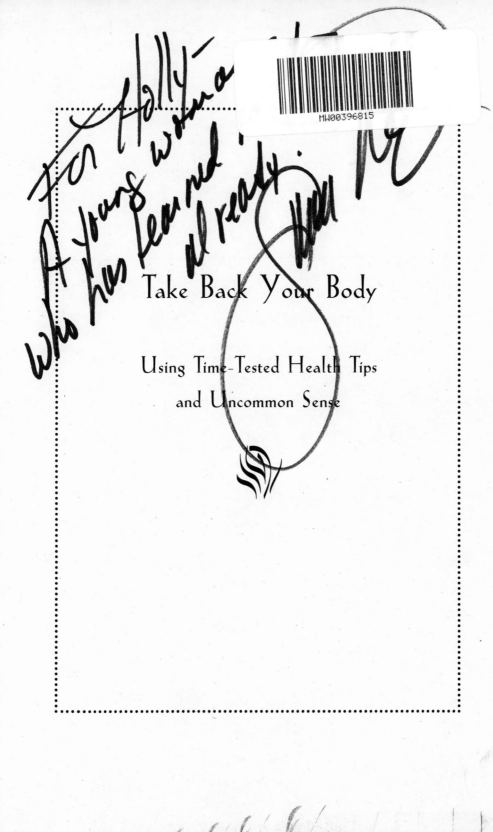

*For Holly—
A yours worm a
who has learned it already.*

Take Back Your Body

Using Time-Tested Health Tips
and Uncommon Sense

Take Back Your Body

Using Time-Tested Health Tips and Uncommon Sense

Susan E. Mead, M.H.

Cover design: F + P Graphic Design, Ft. Collins, CO
Illustrator: E.P. Puffin & Company, Denver, CO
Interior design: WESType Publishing Services, Inc., Boulder, Colorado

Library of Congress Cataloging 2008909545

ISBN 978-0-9822234-0-6 (HB)
ISBN 978-0-6152495-8-2 (P)

Sage&Savvy
PUBLISHING

Mead, Susan E., 1958-
   Take Back Your Body
   1. Health care   2. Nutrition   3. Women Studies

www.SageandSavvyPublishing.com

Printed in Canada

This book is not for those who *need*
the information, but for those who *want* it—
want it enough to do whatever it takes to...

Take Back Your Body

Contents

Chapter Three: How Sex and Meditation Can Get You to the Same Place— And Other Lifestyle Tips   103

Chapter Four: My Favorite Herbs for Healing and Prevention   157

Acknowledgments

Two words I heartily avoid are always and never. That being said, I laugh to myself at the thought of ever being able to create a book alone; anything which makes it to publication has many midwives. The teachers who have gifted me with their knowledge, support, encouragement, love, and gentle kicks in the bum include, but are not limited to, the following:

Herbal Medicine and Ayurveda

My very first teacher of herbs was my grandmother, Esther Mead, who told stories of her mother, my great-grandmother, using herbal teas to help the railroad workers whom she cooked for as a way to respectably get out West in the 1800's. Donald Yance, author of *Herbal Medicine, Healing and Cancer* taught me the value of combining left-brain education with a loving heart; thank you, Donnie, for showing me the true meaning of humility. I am also greatly indebted to Rosita Arvigo, Cascade Anderson Geller, Donna Wild, Pati Caputto, Jill Stansbury, Deepak Chopra, M.D., John Douillard, Terry Willard, Mary Bove, Aviva Romm, Robert Roundtree, M.D., Roy Upton, David Winston, Michael Tierra, Jonathon Treasure, Deborah Frances, Amanda Mcquade Crawford, David Hoffman, Susun Weed, David Simon, M.D., Kerry Bone, Angela Hywood, Paul Bergner, Brigitte Mars, Chancel Cabrerra, Rachel Lord, Peter Holmes, and every valued client since 1996. Those who seek my help have taught me more than years of book-learning. Special thanks to Kenyon Keily, my beloved mentor, teacher and friend for nearly 20 years.

Modern Medicine

Since some physicians still assume that herbalists have a third-eye growing out of their heads, I feel blessed to have many of them as friends, mentors and colleagues. They include Mike Fangman, MD, Miho Scott, M.D., Bev Donnelly, MD, Susan Kozak, MD and the entire team at The Women's Clinic, Robert Roundtree, M.D., Deepak Chopra, M.D., and David Simon, M.D. I have also learned a great deal from Christiane Northurp, M.D., and acknowledge her for being a trailbreaker in holistic health. I am indebted to all of you—for your many lessons and especially for having an open mind. I am particularly grateful to Jacqueline Fields, M.D., my personal physician and long-time supporter.

Yoga

My first and forever-treasured teacher, Chris Lee, whom I studied with multiple times a week for 12 years, has my love and respect. Other high-impact teachers include: Klara Roupp, Judith Lasater, Stacey Swerer, Jane Houck, Carrie McElwee, Zett Amora, Rodney Yee, John Friend, Tomi Simpson, Erich Schiffmann, Gary Craftsow, Jeanne Manchester, and every student I've had the pleasure of having in class.

Writing and Publishing

Writing comes easily for me; editing, polishing and getting to print requires many members of a beautifully orchestrated team. Judith Briles, you head this list for a reason; many blessings to you, not just for your valuable help and guidance—but for believing in me. John Maling, editor extraordinaire, has my gratitude for helping me hone this craft. Additional thanks to Ronnie Moore, Rebecca Finkle, Bobbi Shupe, Margueritte Meier, Janice Hoffman, Sue Sell, Maureen Morris, Anne Lamott and of course, Natalie Goldberg. Though it's been years since I've had the pleasure of connecting with Britt Tippins, she has my thanks for being a great book doctor, as well as my first literary agent.

Life and More

Some family we are born into; other family members are chosen. At the top of my list of chosen family is Elisabeth Reinersmann, my spiritual rudder for 12+ years. My sister, Sarah Mead and my mother, Shirley Mead, were the first in my family of origin to guide me with proper English (most of the time), writing and more. Thank you for loving me through it all. Learning about life has been harder than learning about writing. For these important lessons, I thank Mary Siebe, Diane Fassel, Anne Wilson-Schaef, Kandy Moore, Justin Jones, Shelley Kerr, Rene Clements, Tom Byington, John Motl, M.D., Val Macri-Lind, Barb Brown, Maggie, and Mitch. You have all offered amazing support and education over the years. My darling husband, Webb Jones, deserves many kudos for 11+ years of mostly-silent, Gibraltar-sized support which hasn't wavered. You are my rock.

And then there's office family who have contributed greatly to this labor of love and steadfast belief that helping others heal is why I am on the Earth. Colleen Fine, my Public Relations Director, friend, cheerleader and chick consultant. May God bless you for all you do to help me put one step in front of the other—in a pair of great-looking boots, no less. Sally Castner is a heart of gold that beats regularly in my office, with or without her presence and Vicki Dunn initiated the demise of my being "The Long Ranger." Vicki convinced me 10 or so years ago that I needed an assistant, even though I wasn't paying myself since the practice always needed it more.

But I never worked for free; my clients gave me many lessons, gratitude and love through their dedication to their own health and their smiles of success when they came back. Working for so long without being paid was perfect; it taught me how very little my value was, and is, about how much money I make.

And finally, I acknowledge my greatest teacher—and daughter—Miranda Coy Mead. This "old soul" came into my world on January 11, 1984 and has never ceased to amaze me with her lessons of love, acceptance and awareness. For this reason, and so many others, this book is dedicated to her as the most amazing gift I could receive in this lifetime. Thank you for loving me through the ugly times, and more than anything—thank you for believing in me, Miranda. Especially when I couldn't believe in myself.

*A note on professional designations

I would make a lot of mistakes if I tried to include the proper designations after each of my teachers' names. I thought about leaving off M.D., as well, but let's face it— a mainstream herbalist needs all the credibility she can get. Therefore, I did include that designation (hopefully) with the names of physicians. This *in no way diminishes* the deep respect I have for all those who help others heal—regardless of formal education, money or letters after their names.

Let it be said here, and understood throughout this book, that any insights or helpful hints are due to my many and valued teachers. The mistakes are mine.

Preface

When I was pregnant with my only biological child, Miranda, I thought nine and a half months was a long time to wait for a nine and a half pound baby. But more than two decades later, it doesn't surprise me that it would take nearly nine years to birth a book. Just like many of life's challenges, it's easy to see in hindsight how perfect the end result is—regardless of the snags along the way. If nothing else, *Take Back Your Body* has taught me the meaning of "In God's time, not mine."

The structure of this book, with most of the numbered tips being fewer than 500 words, is designed to allow you to drop in for a few minutes—whether sitting on the throne or waiting for baseball practice to end. I know you're busy and I know that taking back your body is easier said than done in the 21st century. Though I fervently hope you'll find renewed dedication to your own health and sanity, I also want you to be gentle with yourself. There are a lot of "shoulds" out there and I don't want this book to become one of them. Instead, use it for solace in a way-too-fast-and-crazy world. You **can** *Take Back Your Body*, and it works best one step at a time—with a treat after each step. Just remember that a treat doesn't necessarily have to be a hot fudge sundae.

I encourage you to pay special attention to The Quick Six in Appendix E—especially if you're just not finding the time yet to implement many of these tips. The Appendices in the back of the book go into greater detail about certain topics that felt too cumbersome in this format, or didn't fit elsewhere.

Though I had a different working title for the first seven years of this writing project, the title *Take Back Your*

Body has even more significance for me after losing a precious friend, Debrah Rafel Osborn, to one of the bacteria that no longer respond to antibiotics—which she picked up in a hospital during "routine surgery."

Though I have respect for physicians and enjoy working with them, I am gravely concerned about modern health care. It appears to be more about money and profit through "curing," and less about prevention and healing—both of which are often free or very inexpensive. Just because we have access to certain drugs and invasive screening procedures and treatments, doesn't mean we should use them—especially without carefully weighing the costs. And I'm not just talking about money.

Whenever you're told to get a biopsy, schedule surgery or take pharmaceutical or over-the-counter drugs, first remember the credo of Hippocrates, the father of modern medicine: "First, Do No Harm." Ask about alternatives for a diagnostic procedure or treatment which concerns you. Less invasive choices usually exist, often without negative side-effects. It's up to YOU to ask, and to take back responsibility for your body which usually heals itself beautifully—when given the proper tools.

Due to the length of gestation for this book, and my lessons along the way, there are not as many specific references as there would be if I was starting the project now. However, I have provided many URL's for websites and research papers, and a list of books and articles listed in the Bibliography; I encourage you to dig deeper for more information on topics of interest.

Frankly, after nearly 13 years in private practice, it's difficult to sort out the origins of each tidbit. But what I can tell you is, they work, and they are a testimony to my greatest teachers of herbal medicine—my clients. Their names have been changed, but their lessons are threaded throughout this book. Feel free to provide *your* feedback via my web site at *www.SusanEMead.com*.

Susan E. Mead, M.H.
Steamboat Springs, Colorado
Fall 2008

Introduction

"And finally the day will come when the risk it takes
to remain tight in the bud will be more painful
than the risk it takes to blossom."

Anais Nin

Welcome to a simpler path.

I am not a physician, I am not a scientist, I am not a guru. I am a premenopausal woman, herbalist, mom, yoga teacher, spouse and recovering workaholic. Formerly part of the business world for nearly 20 years, I went back to school in 1994, and have been practicing integrative medicine since 1996 as a Master Herbalist. This book contains the basic health principles that I share with my clients and am now offering to you. The most powerful tools in my tackle box are simple: healthy and tasty food choices, moderate exercise, stress reduction and Mother Nature's amazing plants. Ironically, while these healing tools are inexpensive, they are sometimes challenging to sort through and incorporate into very busy lives. That's what this book is all about—helping you simplify the complex maze we now call health care. Redefining health care through self care, you're going to learn some things that will rock your world. Let's go.

Why We Feel Like Slackers

My friend and colleague, Jim, used to give me a hard time about why I was consistently stressed out when I went to see him for acupuncture. "Gee, Susan, do you think you have to eat well, exercise regularly and meditate just to be a good role model for your clients?" he'd ask me. "Well...yes," I responded. "I do." His large belly jiggled as he laughed, saying "Hell, I'd have to charge extra for that!"

I took several pulse diagnosis classes from this highly-talented practitioner who taught me much; but I never forgot his comment about being a good role model after he dropped dead of a heart attack at age 50.

Sad, but true, Jim is not alone. Physicians have some of the highest suicide, alcoholism and divorce rates, often due to practicing very little self care. Though far from perfect myself, I do consider it my moral responsibility to walk my talk as best I can. In addition to the fact that these choices make my present life much more enjoyable, how else could I offer you hope that moving from health care to self care is possible?

The reason most people slack off on healthy living is because it has become so damn complicated, time-consuming and expensive. Many have bought the myth that money and possessions are king; that we are somehow "less than" those who have a more prestigious job, luxurious home or newer car. But do you truly believe you will lie on your death bed, knowing that the end of this precious life is near, and wish you had worked more hours or made more money? When priorities and actions are not in alignment with your values, it's time for a life assessment. Or a kick in the pants.

This is why people seek my help as an herbalist. It may be diverticulitis or menopause or cancer that prompted the phone call, but the illness is often a physical manifestation of a greater imbalance. Watching those in need light up, when they become empowered to create healthy change for themselves, is deeply gratifying—and fosters a growing passion in me to help others.

But this is not about me, or anyone, having all the answers. Your own best health care practitioner is *you* because you know your body in ways that no physician or herbalist can. In fact, a significant part of my role is to remind you of what you already know. You already know you should eat better, exercise more (or start), grab a few minutes of quiet time daily, and love your life along with the people in it. But somehow along the way of Big Macs, cell phones and stressful jobs, your health has been put on hold. Welcome to America.

Big-Picture Health & Healing

Health and healing doesn't mean curing one symptom or disease at a time, while ignoring the rest of your body and the rest of your life. Instead it means creating a foundation of health by eating nutritious and delicious food, exercising regularly, establishing a meditation or relaxation practice, and utilizing Mother Nature's greatest gift—the healing power of plants. Without this foundation of vibrant health, your body will be more susceptible to breaking down in disease, just like a building crumbles without the proper foundation. But unlike buildings, your body has an incredible ability to heal itself—even after years of abuse. With consistent implementation of the simple tips included here, you will feel and see phenomenal improvements in your health.

These suggestions, along with detailed instructions, will help you make some adjustments to the way you live in order to squeeze the juice out of each precious day. Achieving overall physical and mental well-being can be done quite simply, with a few changes in your daily routine. What you eat and the way you eat, how you shop, how you move your body, how you interact with others—it all contributes to the health of your body, mind and soul.

But don't worry; I won't ask you to rearrange your entire life. Instead, these brief tips will remind you to get back to what you already know is the right path. You will also learn some new things you never dreamed could positively impact your health, like the fact that eating *more* quality fats can drastically reduce your sugar cravings while increasing your feeling of being satisfied. And yes, the pounds will drop.

The focus here is how to make sense of what you already know. Perhaps even more important, you'll learn about critical details—like *how* to get more fruits and vegetables into your diet, rather than just a reminder that you need to eat more of them.

Big Bang for Your Investment

Are you interested in looking better, feeling healthier, loving more deeply and having time for what's truly important? If the answer is yes, but you don't have the time and energy for a major life make-over, you've chosen wisely. I guarantee these health tips won't take a lot of time and won't cost much, either. Did you know that certain herbs and spices available at the grocery store can actually help prevent diseases like cancer and heart disease? Did you know about the ones that can help you have a better love life? These simple tips are easy to implement, but I'm also asking you to re-think your relationship with food, your body and much more.

I struggled to keep the chapter on herbs short and simple—a challenge, since I have over 180 to choose from in my herbal dispensary. Ideally, you will receive referrals from your friends to find a top-notch herbalist, or another health care practitioner, who uses a sound foundation of nutritional support and lifestyle choices to provide a customized approach just for you. But in the meantime, the herbal medicine tips in Chapter Four will give you a quick start.

If you need even more of a shortcut to learn about moving from health care to self care, see The Quick Six in Appendix E for the down and dirty tidbits. It's for those of you who have good intentions, but will never read most of this book.

Time-Savers, Too!

Most of us feel time-deprived and yet the average American adult spends four to five hours a day watching TV. No judgment here; just looking for ways to help you return to balance. It's taken you years to get to this place, so give yourself the gift of doing this gradually. Start with implementing just one change—today. Perhaps you can incorporate one or two quick tips each week to remind yourself that creating and maintaining health is an important and evolving process. Keep this book in the bathroom for a time-saving reminder if you're a multi-tasker. You'll find most of these tips to be 500 words or less.

Rather than feeling guilty about not doing this perfectly, celebrate small changes. In addition to being alive longer to enjoy your friends, children and grandchildren, you'll be active and fit enough to squeeze the juice out of life! Perhaps most important of all, you'll be setting a great example for future generations. Teenagers have taught me tons about my illusion of control, reminding me that the best sermon is a good example. I invite you to *be* that example.

Another valued teacher of mine is my friend, Melanie Mills, who is an awesome public speaker who has often told her audiences the story of talking with my daughter Miranda about her hamsters. Melanie was intrigued with all the "tricks" Miranda had the hamsters doing—from bungee jumping to racecar driving—but what captured her interest the most was watching those hamsters run around in their wheels. She said this is exactly the way her life felt; like a hamster running as fast as he could, but getting nowhere. This feeling is not exclusive to Melanie—or to you. Most of us have succumbed to the great American way of fast food, fast cars and working ourselves to death, in order to buy more toys or have the illusion of security. My bet is you're searching for more. And less.

If you're like me, and many I have worked with, you're ready to get off that hamster's wheel. You're researching "alternative" medicine, experimenting with herbs or getting an occasional massage to unwind. You're stressed, tired, perhaps menopausal—and at your wits end trying to sift through the myriad of information about how to improve your health and regain control of your life. What are you finding? Overwhelming options and no time or energy to pursue them? Do you keep searching, hoping that someone can simplify all of this for you?

Take a deep breath and repeat after me: there is hope. Creating a healthy lifestyle does not mean you need to quit your job, take a six-month course on macrobiotic cooking, spend an hour every day meditating and read 20 pages in a book every time you want to take an herb safely. What it does mean is that you have to get real. What you've been doing isn't working. You know the rest: if you do what you've always done, you'll get what you've always gotten. Sick, tired, depressed, and cranky. Maybe chunky, too.

Receiving More While Doing Less

Considering how full our lives are, I knew these tips needed to be short and easily mastered. My goal is for you to move from health care to self care, using affordable and simple tips that have worked beautifully for hundreds of my health-conscious clients. There are short suggestions on how to heal your relationship with food (#1) and serve a fabulous green vegetable in five minutes that your kids will actually eat (#3). You'll find tips on how to "medi-tate" while you're driving (#52), practice yoga while watching TV (#27), and start the day with three servings of fruits that are delicious and easy (#4).

You'll find quick tips on the one herb we all need at some point for our immune system (# 52), which menopause herbs are most effective (# 54), and which herbs help almost everyone with seasonal allergies (#53). Certainly, I must cau-tion you: it is always best to consult a qualified and respected herbalist before experimenting on your own. It's a must if you're on any prescription or over-the-counter drugs.

Your pharmacist may be a good resource regarding potential herb-drug interactions as well as drug-drug interactions which are far more common. Always pay close attention to your body when trying a new herb or pharmaceutical drug. Headaches, dizziness or nausea may be signaling an adverse reaction—which is rare with herbs, especially if you're not on any pharmaceuticals.

Now take a deep breath, drink a sip of tea or wine, and drop into these quick tips as time permits. They're perfect while waiting for the oil to be changed in your car or for your child to finish soccer practice. If you're short on time, skim through the table of contents for the topics currently in your face, rather than reading each tip in order. Either way, know that I care.

My clients have taught me much more about healing than I've learned in years of formal education. Let's continue to teach each other and express gratitude for all the ways we enjoy our health now, while improving our future.

Chapter One

Food as Medicine— With a Sensual and Savory Experience on Top

"Let food be your medicine and your medicine be your food."

Hippocrates

J anice, a 39 year-old mother of three, had been a client of mine for six months when she invited me to visit her family for a food overhaul. I had offered this service a few weeks prior in my monthly newsletter as a way to create a fresh start on better nutrition.

Fortunately, the children and their father also wanted a healthy pantry and better alternatives to their family favorites: Pop-Tarts, cold cereal, Hamburger Helper and Oreos. They were excited to learn that bacon and eggs are healthier than cold breakfast cereals; a dish made of organic hamburger, brown rice pasta and no-sugar marinara sauce out of a jar tastes delicious; and cookies made at home with wholesome ingredients are healthier, taste better, and are less expensive than those from the grocery store.

1. Heal Your Relationship with Food

Let's start by understanding how you relate to food. Those who know me believe I'm one of the healthiest eaters on the planet, but I certainly have my weak moments; they've never seen me gobbling down leftover Easter candy in a moment of emotional need while visiting my mom. Healing your relationship with food can be a difficult and lifelong process if you received mixed messages early in life.

This is clearly not a quick-fix issue. However, I've worked with many clients who are living proof it can be done. Eating disorders can include bulimia (binging and purging), anorexia (not eating much at all), and plain old vanilla overeating. If you believe you're suffering from an eating disorder, please get help. Find a therapist with experience in this area and invest in your healing. Group therapy can be especially beneficial for resolving these issues.

Healing your relationship with food is best accomplished in stages. At first you might cut back on sodas. Then, after a few weeks or months, try eliminating them altogether. Regular soda is poisonous, and diet soda even more so (see #15). Next you might cut back on junk food. It will likely still be part of your daily diet, but, hopefully, significantly less. After several more weeks or months, you may decide to start buying organic produce (#16), and then make the commitment to purchase free-range, hormone-free, antibiotic-free meat and poultry. When I reached this stage, I stopped ordering red meat when dining out since restaurants rarely offer organic meats. I make one exception, however: Morton's Steakhouse. When my husband and I splurge at Morton's, I just love to break this guideline. It's the best steak ever—and I grew up in Nebraska!

My latest stage of nutritional healing resulted from an unwanted and frustrating gift. After turning 40, my metabolism changed; I gained 15 pounds in three months even though I hadn't changed my eating or exercise habits. It took me two years of killing myself with martial arts training and extra weekly miles of running to realize that changing my eating habits was the only solution. I was terrified. After healing many of my food issues, I still thought that deprivation and dieting were necessary to lose weight, which I swore I would never do again. But I had to accept the fact that exercise alone (even fifteen hours a week of it), was not going to budge that extra weight.

My *aha* moment came watching The Oprah Show. Dr. Phil McGraw was on, talking about "Getting Real" about weight loss. I knew there was still junk to cut out of my diet, and I knew the way to do it was to focus on what I wanted to eat rather than the food I wanted to eliminate. I decided walnuts and macadamia nuts taste almost as good as potato chips, and as a bonus they have more omega-3 essential fatty acids (EFA's) than most other foods. I released most of the extra weight by cutting way back on sugar and refined carbohydrates—both of which contribute to all Western diseases. More later on weight loss (#8).

2. Eat Your Fruits and Veggies

Remember what your grandmother used to say? "Eat your fruits and vegetables!" Well, she was right. For your health, if you do nothing other than consume five to seven servings of fresh fruits and veggies each day, you'll be way ahead of most Americans. The majority of us consume only one or two servings a day—if you count orange juice. No time, you say? Not a fast enough food for our fast-paced society? You'll be amazed at how quick and easy fruit and veggies are if you think ahead a little.

When you know it's going to be one of those jam-packed days, take five minutes in the morning or the night before to "bag it". Cut up a few of your favorite veggies and toss them into a zip-lock bag—or better yet, a reusable storage container. Choose from red and green peppers, celery, broccoli, cauliflower, carrots, or whatever makes your heart sing—and pump. Many of these are now available in organic bite-sized pieces at your local market or health food store.

Keeping a bag of veggies ready to go helps you make healthier choices when time is short. For an even greater incentive, many articles point to a significantly lower risk of cancer for those who enjoy four to eight servings of fruits and vegetables each day. See *breastcancer.org* and *medicalnewstoday.com* for more specifics. Now, let's explore *how* to incorporate that much produce into your daily diet—with ease.

Starting your day with a Smoothie (#4) provides two to three servings of fruit before you walk out the door. If lunch looks like a fantasy, take your baggie with veggies and a handful of nuts with you to eat in the car. When possible, find a nearby park for a few relaxing minutes with your noontime meal. Even if you're eating on the run or in the car that day, these choices will be infinitely healthier (and hundreds of calories less) than a burger, fries, and a soda.

If lunches are your best business opportunity, necessitating restaurant meals on a regular basis, choose a healthy entree with a salad. Ask your server how the main dish is prepared and the type of oil used. If you're low-key about this—and tip well—the server and the person you're having lunch with will learn something from you rather than label you as some type of health nut.

Sometimes when lunching out, I'll ask the server to bring me just a whole carrot in addition to the salad. No peeling or chopping—just bring me a clean carrot. They occasionally look at me strangely, but I'll get one to two servings of carrots that way and often the server won't even charge me. Since carrots are an alkaline food they provide a bonus: they help mitigate excess stomach acids caused by stress.

An afternoon snack of an orange, an apple with a thin slice of Romano cheese or a small handful of nuts or seeds will keep blood sugar levels even and your crankiness at bay. The nuts are especially good for those who need protein to minimize the mid-afternoon energy slump. If you choose an orange for your snack, it will likely just sit on your desk as a guilty reminder that the vending machine candy bar is easier—unless you section it the night before.

Now for dinner. You've had three fruits and two veggies; only two more to go. The more I understand the

benefits of greens, the more I enjoy and recommend salads. Mine at home are nothing fancy because if I have to
take the time to cut up five different things, it's not going
to happen. Often I'll just tear off some leaf lettuce and
then add to it the "Spring Mix" available in most grocery
stores. This combination of healthy greens usually contains arugula, radicchio, frisee, baby red chard, mizuna,
and baby spinach.

According to Susun Weed, herbalist extraordinaire,
cooking greens with some quality fat helps break down
the nutrients from the start, making them easier to digest
in the sluggish months of winter. But during the rest of
the year, drizzling some olive oil on your greens is enough
to start that break-down of nutrients. Almost all prepared
salad dressings are bad news, so play it safe by requesting
oil and vinegar when in a restaurant. Dried cranberries,
raisins, or pumpkin seeds make tasty salad additions
at home.

Finally, if you prepare The Best Broccoli Ever (#3),
which takes only five minutes, or cut up jicama or red
pepper to put on top of your salad, you're up to seven
fruits and veggies for that day—congratulations!

Susan's Simple Tip
What's a serving, you ask? Keep it simple: the
amount of food that fits in the palm of your hand;
typically about ½ cup.

3. The Best Broccoli Ever!

Andrew Weil, M.D. has written many helpful books on how to enjoy good health. In Weil's first book, *Eight Weeks to Optimum Health*, he provided a recipe for the best broccoli I've ever tasted. The key is peeling the outside of the stalks to remove the bitterness. It's so healthy and nutritious, we eat it at least once a week. Easy to prepare and with a minimum of ingredients, your whole family will love it—guaranteed. If you have children who complain about things being too spicy, just omit the red-pepper flakes. This broccoli recipe will quickly become part of your weekly repertoire since it cooks in only five minutes, tastes great, easily fulfills a veggie serving (about ½ cup) and has garlic for your immune system. Yum!

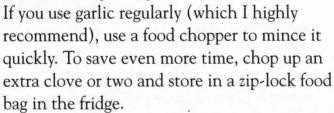

Susan's Simple Tip

If you use garlic regularly (which I highly recommend), use a food chopper to mince it quickly. To save even more time, chop up an extra clove or two and store in a zip-lock food bag in the fridge.

The Best Broccoli Ever

1 large bunch broccoli
1 T. extra-virgin olive oil
salt to taste
several cloves garlic, chopped
red-pepper flakes to taste (optional)

Trim the bottoms of the broccoli stalks and discard. Cut off the main stem of each stalk, peel it with a vegetable peeler and cut the flesh into bite-sized chunks. Separate the head of broccoli into bite-sized pieces. Wash the broccoli in cold water, drain, and place in a pot with ¼ cup cold water, olive oil, garlic, and salt to taste. Add a pinch or more of the hot red-pepper flakes if you want a spicy dish.

Bring to a boil, cover tightly, and let steam until the broccoli is bright green and very crunchy-tender; *no more* than five minutes. Remove with a slotted spoon and serve at once. You can also add the broccoli (with any remaining liquid) to cooked pasta, seasoning it with freshly-grated parmesan or Romano cheese if you like.

4. The Ultimate Smoothie

With the recent introduction of smoothie/juice bars in the U.S., many have discovered a delicious way to enjoy more fruit. But at $4 each, you could spend $120 a month on breakfast alone—for one person. These expensive smoothies also have more sugar than you want. Chances are you have a blender at home that is capable of mixing up more than margaritas. It can also help you include quality yogurt (i.e. whole, organic, and plain) and coconut milk in your diet. They both add the consistency of ice cream to your smoothie and provide great nutrition. I also suggest adding ground flax seeds, especially for menopausal women. This addition is a healthy alternative to Premarin (made from mare's urine) which is often prescribed to ease change-of-life symptoms. The essential fatty acids in flax seeds not only balance hormones, but provide necessary omega-3 oils and added fiber. Here's my basic smoothie recipe; feel free to get creative.

Susan's Simple Tip
If mornings are especially busy, double or triple the recipe and pour off an extra glass for the next day or two. Not quite as fresh, but it's worth the compromise if it keep's you from stopping for fast food.

The Ultimate Smoothie

8-12 ounces of water (no calories and less sugar
    than using juice or milk)
1 cup frozen blueberries, strawberries, cranberries—
    or any other berries you like
½-1 banana at any stage of ripeness (optional)
4-6 T. whole, plain, organic yogurt
¼ can of coconut milk
1-2 T. ground flax seeds for essential fatty acids (#13)
1 t.-1 T. high-vitamin cod liver oil (lemon-flavor
    optional)
1 raw egg (optional, but recommended)
½ sheet Nori seaweed torn into pieces (optional
    for thyroid support)
¼-½ t. raw honey if sweetener is needed (likely not)

    Blend until smooth and sip with a straw if you
don't want to take a smoothie mustache to work.
This is an easy and delicious way to get two to
three servings of fruit in your daily diet. It satisfies
your hunger even after an aggressive morning
workout, and stays with you right up until lunch
due to the fat and protein in the egg, coconut milk
and yogurt.

5. Lessons from the Past

In addition to teachers like Susun Weed, Donald Yance, Christiane Northrup, Sally Fallon and Deepak Chopra I've been honored to learn from in person, there are physicians and nutritionists from the 19th century who have greatly impacted my work; especially the eclectic physicians who employed whatever was found to be beneficial to their patients, including herbs (eclectic being derived from the Greek word "eklego", meaning "to choose from").

Eclectic doctors practiced with a philosophy of "alignment with nature," learning from and using concepts from other schools of medical thought, including Native American medicine. They opposed the techniques of bleeding, chemical purging and the use of mercury compounds common among the "conventional" doctors of that time. Instead, they espoused simple and wholesome food choices such as raw milk, quality beef and poultry, fish, fruits and vegetables, cod liver oil and fermented foods and/or beverages—often raw apple cider vinegar. Ahead of their time, these pioneers were often verbally stoned for their ideas which have now proven to be correct.

Raw honey, high-vitamin cod liver oil, raw apple cider vinegar and organic butter (preferably from raw milk) are "Super Foods" with special nutritional benefits—foods which can often replace expensive medications and supplements. To keep this simple, I've listed the basic benefits of regularly consuming these foods—listed and described below—with my encouragement to research further and make your own decisions.

Susan's Simple Tip

For those interested in the benefits of traditional diets, I suggest researching *WestonAPrice.org*. You will see many references to the Weston Price Foundation in this chapter. I find their website to be the very best for uncommon sense regarding nutrition, and they are not trying to sell supplements or anything else to you—other than membership which is a bargain.

Cod Liver Oil

There is hardly a disease on the books that does not respond well to a protocol that includes cod liver oil, not just infections but also chronic modern diseases like heart disease and cancer. Cod liver oil provides vitamin D to help build strong bones in children and prevent osteoporosis in adults. The fatty acids in cod liver oil are also essential for the development of the brain and nervous system, helping to prevent learning disabilities. Cod liver oil greatly improves heart function to prevent CHD (coronary heart disease), and can even be used to treat it in advanced stages, after a patient has had a heart attack or heart surgery.

Obesity, hypertension, stroke, adult onset diabetes and insulin resistance all appear to be minimized with regular consumption of cod liver oil. See *WomentoWomen.com* for more information on insulin resistance. In numerous studies, the elongated omega-3 fats found in cod liver oil have been shown to improve brain function, memory, bone health, stress response, immune response, allergies, asthma, and learning and behavioral disorders, including bipolar syndrome and manic-depression. The website found at *WestonAPrice.org* also lists detailed information about cod liver oil.

Fermented Foods, Including Apple Cider Vinegar

In earlier times, people knew how to preserve vegetables for long periods without the use of freezers or canning machines through the process of lacto-fermentation. The ancient Greeks understood that important chemical changes take place during this type of fermentation. Their name for this change was "alchemy."

Like the fermentation of dairy products, preservation of vegetables and fruits by lacto-fermentation has numerous advantages beyond those of simple preservation. The proliferation of lactobacilli in fermented vegetables enhances their digestibility and increases vitamin levels. These beneficial organisms produce numerous helpful enzymes as well as antibiotic and anti-carcinogenic substances.

In Europe the principle lacto-fermented food is sauerkraut, made from cabbage. Cucumbers, beets and turnips are also traditional European foods for lacto-fermentation. In Russia and Poland one finds pickled green tomatoes, peppers and lettuces. Lacto-fermented foods form part of Asian cuisines as well. American tradition includes many types of relishes—corn relish, cucumber relish, watermelon rind—all of which are lacto-fermented products.

Start simply by including just one or two fermented foods into your daily diet. A teaspoon of raw (i.e. non-pasteurized) apple cider vinegar in glass of water will not only provide the health benefits listed above, but has been proven to assist long-term weight loss and will often prevent a blossoming headache—even a migraine. Another easy way to include fermented foods in your diet is through a delicious drink called kombucha. Found in health food stores in a variety of flavors, this is an easy way to strengthen your body's defenses—especially your immune response which needs healthy bacteria called microflora to function well.

Scientists and doctors today are mystified by the proliferation of new viruses—not only the deadly AIDS virus but the whole gamut of human viruses that seem to be associated with everything from chronic fatigue to cancer and arthritis. Could it be that in abandoning the ancient practice of lacto-fermentation and our insistence that everything in our diet be pasteurized, we have compromised the health of our intestinal flora and made ourselves vulnerable to legions of pathogenic microorganisms?

Raw Dairy

Through our fear of bacteria (justified, given the cleanliness of most commercial dairies), we have come to believe that pasteurization is good and necessary—but it also destroys many of our food's nutrients. Though countries like India have enjoyed the benefits of raw dairy for years, it's questionable whether we humans truly need dairy in our diets. I suggest organic butter and whole, plain yogurt (both milk products), but I'm intrigued that we are the only mammal that consumes milk itself after weaning. Do we need it to be healthy? I think not, especially if most of the nutrients have been destroyed by heating via pasteurization. Learn more at *rawmilk.org* and decide for yourself.

Butter—It's Healthy!

Heart disease was rare in America at the turn of the century. Between 1920 and 1960, the incidence of heart disease rose precipitously, making it America's number one killer. During the same period, butter consumption plummeted from 18 pounds per person per year to four. It doesn't take a Ph.D. in statistics to conclude that butter is not a cause of heart disease. Actually, butter contains many nutrients that protect us from heart disease.

First among these is vitamin A which is needed for the health of the thyroid and adrenal glands, both of which play a role in maintaining the proper functioning of the heart and cardiovascular system. Abnormalities of the heart and larger blood vessels occur in babies born to vitamin A deficient mothers. Butter is America's best and most easily absorbed source of vitamin A. Surprised?

Butter contains lecithin, a substance that assists in the proper assimilation and metabolism of cholesterol and other fat constituents. It also contains a number of antioxidants that protect against the kind of free-radical damage that weakens the arteries. Vitamin A and vitamin E, both found in butter, play a strong anti-oxidant role in the body. Butter is also a rich source of selenium, a vital anti-oxidant known to help prevent cancer.

In addition, butter is a good dietary source of cholesterol which is a potent anti-oxidant that floods into the

blood when we take in too many harmful free-radicals—
usually from damaged and rancid fats in margarine and
highly processed vegetable oils. A Medical Research Coun-
cil survey showed that men eating butter ran half the risk
of developing heart disease as those using margarine.

Susan's Simple Tip
For more details regarding butter as a health food
and other radical notions, do a search on "butter"
at *WestonAPrice.org*.

6. Soy Alert

Perhaps you've been waiting for me to promote soy products. A few years ago, I would have; but when we know better, we do better. After a great deal of research, I've learned to reach back a couple of generations to find the common sense nutrition our ancestors thrived on. Perhaps Asian people maintain their health with *minimally-processed* soy foods by using them in combination with many vegetables and fish. But recent studies express concern for Westerners who believe our processed version of soy is nutritious. Do an internet search on "soy concerns" using *www.fda.gov*.

Part of the problem lies with "foods" like soy hot dogs, soy cheese and highly-processed soy protein powder; they look nothing like the actual soy bean. Just as whole wheat's excessive processing destroys its nutritional value, the soy bean's nutrients can be destroyed by adding chemicals to make it palatable to Western taste buds. Reported on the Weston A. Price website are these concerns with soy:

◆ High levels of phytic acid in soy reduce assimilation of calcium, magnesium, copper, iron and zinc. Phytic acid in soy is not neutralized by ordinary preparation methods such as soaking, sprouting and long, slow cooking. High phytate diets have caused growth problems in children.

◆ Trypsin inhibitors in soy interfere with protein digestion and may cause pancreatic disorders. In test animals, soy-containing trypsin inhibitors caused stunted growth.

◆ Vitamin Bone2 analogs in soy are not absorbed and actually increase the body's requirement for Bone2.

◆ Soy foods increase the body's requirement for vitamin D.

◆ Processing of soy protein results in the formation of toxic lysinoalanine and highly carcinogenic nitrosamines.

◆ Free glutamic acid or MSG, a potent neurotoxin, is formed during soy food processing and additional amounts are added to many soy foods. Ask to have it left out of your food at Asian restaurants.

◆ Soy foods contain high levels of aluminum which is toxic to the nervous system and the kidneys.

From a clinical perspective, I've seen many clients who have significant digestive problems due to consuming too much *unfermented* soy. As soon as they cut back or eliminate it from their diet, their GI problems disappear. A coincidence? Perhaps, but I think not. The fermented types of soy which are found not to cause digestive problems include miso (a fermented paste used most commonly in soups), tamari soy sauce and tempeh (fermented soybeans pressed into a cake).

You may not feel convinced, but when in doubt, leave it out. There are many other ways to get quality nutrition in the West. But continue to enjoy edamame which is the actual soy bean; they're green and clearly a whole food by their appearance and taste.

7. Take the Fear Out of Fat

Due to heavy marketing by the food industry and choles-terol-lowering-drug companies, Americans have become obsessive about reducing, or even eliminating, fat from the diet. Notice how well it's working; our culture has more problems with obesity than ever before! The sole success of this campaign is in lining the pockets of large food companies and drug companies using faulty evidence from the 1950's. I beg of you—*never buy a low-fat product again.*

Whenever a wholesome product like plain, whole yogurt is made into a low-fat product, something else has to be added to make it taste good. Usually, it's sugar or starchy fillers or both. A small container of low-fat yogurt has 26 grams of sugar. You're much better off buying plain, whole, organic yogurt and mixing in your own fruit—you'll save money, too. I'd rather spend it and my sugar calories on a delicious piece of Godiva chocolate instead.

Even though most people on low-fat diets don't feel healthy or energetic, there's a belief that avoiding fat is the healthy choice. The modern medicine community, junk food industry and the media have done a great job convincing the American public that fats are bad for us, and that vegetable oils are better in their place. Here's a different version of the truth.

◆ In the process of producing vegetable oils, toxic chemicals and high temperatures are used to extract the oil from the seed or bean. This process destroys the nutritional value and

actually turns the oils rancid before you can
bring them home. It's best to eliminate all
vegetable oils: those polyunsaturates that we've
been told are so good for us.

◆ Margarine is an artificial concoction of chemicals
and hydrogenated oils. Legally, it can still contain
some of those poisonous trans fatty acids without
listing them on the ingredients label. Not only
does it lack flavor, but won't even melt on your
toast, indicating an unnatural state.

◆ Butter is a rich source of fat-soluble vitamins A,
D, E, and K. The saturated fat in butter actually
enhances immune function, protects the liver
from toxins, nourishes the heart in times of
stress, and aids in the proper utilization of
omega-3 essential fatty acids.

◆ Coconut and palm oils are rich sources of
saturated fat, especially lauric acid, which has
strong antifungal and antimicrobial properties.
These oils, inappropriately maligned, are
extremely stable and can be used in baking,
frying, sautéing and for making popcorn.

◆ According to a study published in The Lancet
(1994, 344:1195), the fatty acids found in
clogged arteries are mostly unsaturated fats,
not saturated, as we have been led to believe.
For Good News On Saturated Fats, by John
Tierney, see the July 21, 2008 edition of The
New York Times. He is quoting a new report
from The New England Journal of Medicine,
July 17, 2008.

More good news is that consuming enough *quality* fats reduces your cravings for sugar which has many harmful effects on the body, including adding extra pounds. This happened with my body and with many clients; and the physicians I work with confirm these findings. More quality fat in the diet equals fewer sugar cravings.

One of my favorite statistics is about the women of Crete having the lowest incidences of heart disease, diabetes and cancer in the world while they enjoy 50 percent of their calories from good sources of fat. I'm sure part of that statistic has to do with physical exercise, too, but clearly a higher fat diet is not the killer we've been led to believe. Many traditional peoples consume up to 50, 60, even 80 percent of their diets in quality fats.

I'm about to further rock your world with some amazing facts about fat. Part of the following information comes from the cookbook, *Nourishing Traditions* by Sally Fallon. Her 60-page introduction is truly enlightening regarding the "party line" on food and nutrition. This one book will teach you about good nutrition and cooking simultaneously. And, you'll come away with a gnawing sense of being sold a bill of goods about fat—and you have been!

Fallon opens our eyes to the fallacies of politically correct nutrition which is based on the assumption that we should reduce our intake of fats, particularly saturated fats from animal sources. Since the latter also contain cholesterol, they have become the twin villains of the civilized diet. The theory—called the lipid hypothesis— that there is a direct relationship between the amount of saturated fat and cholesterol in the diet and the incidence of coronary heart disease was proposed by a researcher named Ancel Keys in the late 1950's.

A specific link on his conclusions can be found at: *WestonAPrice.org/federalupdate/testimony/comments_dietary guidelinesrep*

Numerous subsequent studies have questioned Keys' data and conclusions, but received little publicity. The vegetable oil and food processing industries which bene-fit most from research that finds fault with competing tra-ditional foods, began promoting and funding further research designed to support the lipid hypothesis. You may be skeptical—I was, too—but consider the following from *Nourishing Traditions*:

◆ Before 1920 coronary heart disease was rare in America, but by the mid-fifties heart disease was the leading cause of death among Americans. Today heart disease causes at least 50% of all US deaths. If, as we have been told, heart disease results from the consumption of saturated fats, you would expect to find an increase in animal fat in the American diet. However, the reverse is true. Between 1910 and 1970, the proportion of traditional animal fat in our diet declined from 83 percent to 62 percent, and butter consumption went from 18 pounds per person per year to four! During the past 80 years, dietary cholesterol intake has increased only one percent. During the same period the percentage of dietary vegetable oils in the form of margarine, shortening and refined oils increased about

400 percent while the consumption of sugar and processed foods increased about 60 percent.

◆ In a multi-year British study involving several thousand men, half were asked to reduce saturated fat and cholesterol in their diets, to stop smoking and to increase the amounts of unsaturated oils such as margarine and vegetable oils—the so called "good" diet. After one year, those on the "good" diet had 100 percent more deaths than those on the "bad" diet, in spite of the fact those men on the "bad" diet continued to smoke!

◆ Mother's milk provides a higher proportion of cholesterol than any other food. It also contains over 50 percent of its calories as fat, much of it saturated fat. Both cholesterol and saturated fat are essential for growth in babies and children, especially the development of the brain. Yet, the American Heart Association is now recommending a low-cholesterol, low-fat diet for children! Commercial formulas are low in saturated fats and soy formulas have no cholesterol. A recent study linked low-fat diets with failure to thrive in children.

◆ The relative good health of the Japanese, who have the longest life span of any nation in the world, is generally attributed to a low-fat diet. Although they do consume few dairy fats, the notion that the Japanese diet is low in fat is a myth. It contains moderate amounts of animal fats from eggs, pork, chicken, beef, seafood and

organ meats. The Japanese probably consume
more cholesterol than most Americans. What
they do *not* consume is a lot of vegetable oil,
white flour, hydrogenated oils and processed food
(although they do eat white rice). The life span
of the Japanese has increased since World War II
with an increase in animal fat and protein in
their diet. And remember—they eat significantly
more vegetables than the average American.

Clearly something is wrong with the theories we read
in the popular press which are used to bolster sales of low-
fat concoctions and cholesterol-free foods. The notion
that saturated fats *per se* cause heart disease as well as cancer is just plain wrong. But it *is* true that some fats are bad
for us. Details about which ones we should avoid follow,
but if you want to keep it really simple, choose the fats
that have been around a long time (butter, nuts, avocados, olive oil, coconut oil, lard, etc.) and avoid the new
kids on the block (hydrogenated oils of any kind and
most polyunsaturated oils).

I'm convinced that part of the reason my grandfather
lived to be 103 and my grandmother made it to 98 is due
to their old-fashioned food choices. I remember them eating meat or fish daily, potatoes or beans, lots of veggies
from the garden, and bacon & eggs on the weekends.
Sounds good, doesn't it?

Good Fats

Monounsaturated Fats—found in olives and olive oil, and
some varieties of nuts (cashews, almonds, and macadamia

nuts) and avocados. These are also found in canola oil which is getting mixed reviews currently, so it's best to use olive oil or butter instead.

These heart-healthy fats actually lower LDL (the "bad" cholesterol) without affecting HDL (the "good" cholesterol) that improves your ratio of total cholesterol to HDL and lowers your triglicerides. Both of those numbers are far more critical than your total cholesterol—see #83 for more specifics.

Cultures using monounsaturated fats as their primary cooking fat (Mediterranean diets) have far less incidence of heart disease and stroke than we do. Some studies also report that monounsaturated fats may protect against cancer. I suggest making olive oil your cooking oil of choice except for baking or cooking at high temperatures. Butter and tropical oils (palm and coconut) work well for baked goods.

Snack on raw seeds or nuts regularly (in small quantities if calories are an issue). I keep raw almonds in a ziplock baggie in my purse at all times; even four or five of these healthy nuts keep blood sugar levels even until your busy life allows a meal. See Appendix B on Digestion for more about hypoglycemia and blood sugar levels.

Omega-3 Essential Fatty Acids (EFA's)—found in salmon, sardines, herring, kippers, mackerel, walnuts, flax seeds, and hemp seeds.

These highly unsaturated fats, known as omega-3's, became the wonder fats of the nineties when studies showed their positive association with lower risk of blood clots, heart arrhythmia, high blood pressure, kidney disease, and cancer. A study in the Journal of the American Medical Association (JAMA) suggests that eating fish rich in omega-3's at least once a week may cut the risk of sudden cardiac death in *half*. They may also help reduce the risk of severe depression, bipolar disorder (manic-depressive disorder) and schizophrenia.

Choose fish at least once or twice a week and add one to two tablespoons of ground flaxseed to your daily diet. You can add the flax to soups, sauces and smoothies, or sprinkle them on salads. Include raw walnuts on a regular basis to improve brain function. Ever notice how they even look like a brain?

Susan's Simple Tip
JAMA (Journal of The American Medical Association) offers many online articles for free. The one I refer to here can be found at: *ama.ama-assn.org/cgi/content/full/295/22/26one3*.

Saturated Fats—found in animal foods such as meats, poultry, whole milk, cream, butter, cheese and egg yolks, as well as palm oil and coconut oil.

This is the rock-your-world part. Based on the data I've reviewed and my own experience with clients, I'm convinced that including some saturated fats is not only acceptable but highly beneficial. Many people in the West suffer needlessly from chronic diseases which could be mitigated with the proper use of what I consider to be high-quality fats, including saturated fats, often lacking in the diets of our low-fat-obsessed world.

I want to emphasize the importance of choosing *quality* animal products without added hormones, antibiotics or anything else Mother Nature doesn't include. Including quality animal fats and eliminating the newfangled oils is a huge step in the health direction. Use organic butter confidently, with the assurance that it is a wholesome food for you and your family; it contains butyric acid, an important anticancer agent.

Regarding the tropical oils such as coconut and palm, they do not contribute to heart disease but have nourished healthy populations for thousands of years. The saturated fat scare has forced manufacturers to abandon these safe and healthy oils in favor of hydrogenated soybean, corn, canola and cottonseed oils which are often poison for us due to their processing. Intuitively, it seems the tropical oils would be best suited to those who live in the tropics, but I have seen no convincing evidence they are harmful for the rest of us, and they are stable at higher heat unlike the highly-touted polyunsaturates.

Bad Fats

Polyunsaturated Fats—found in corn oil, soybean oil, sunflower oil, safflower oil and cottonseed oil, as well as oils used as seasoning such as sesame, walnut, and hazelnut oils. Not only do polyunsaturated fats lower "good" cholesterol along with the "bad", they're also chemically unstable, resulting in toxic compounds that can damage DNA and cell membranes. This can result in a greater chance of cancer and tissue degeneration.

These oils contain omega-6 fatty acids that you need in your diet, but most people overload on omega-6's while skimping on the essential omega-3's. Some experts believe the ideal ratio should be four to one but the average American takes in 20 times more omega-6's than omega-3's. Polyunsaturated fats are ubiquitous in the American diet, so even if you greatly reduce them, you're bound to get enough omega-6's. It's best to avoid most of these, but I do make one exception: dark (roasted) sesame oil. It has an intense taste and it takes a small amount to flavor food. Use a few drops to a teaspoon at most, to season soups and stir-fry at the end of cooking or in a salad dressing. You can use walnut oil or hazelnut oil in small amounts for similar purposes.

Ugly Fats

Trans-Fatty Acids (TFA's)—found in margarine, vegetable shortening, hydrogenated vegetable oils and products made from them. These include nearly all commercial snack foods such as crackers, cakes, cookies, pastries, spreads and some cereals. I call TFA's legal poison. They're created when manufacturers bubble hydrogen through heated polyunsaturated oils in order to make them more stable for frying and to extend shelf life. This is an unnatural process and truly is poison to your body. Not only do TFA's raise LDL ("bad" cholesterol) as saturated fats do, but they also lower HDL ("good" cholesterol). Many experts consider TFA's to be the chief dietary culprit regarding heart attacks.

Eliminate the use of margarine and vegetable shortening (like Crisco), as well as anything deep-fried in restaurants. The oils they use for frying are often used way too long, making them even *more* dangerous. (One more reason to eat wholesome foods at home.) Once you start looking for partially hydrogenated oils on product labels, you'll be amazed at how often you find them. I know it's a challenge, but eliminating these manufactured oils from your diet could be the single greatest thing you do to improve your health long-term.

Susan's Simple Tip

Most grocery stores now carry a pre-made guacamole that is delicious, has no preservatives, and is no more expensive than homemade. Look for it in a box where you find refrigerated salad dressings. This is a very tasty and healthy source of fat. I like to add a bit of fresh lemon juice, Tabasco and sea salt when time permits.

8. Cranberry-Wheatberry Salad

This is another one of Andrew Weil's recipes. If you're still eating wheat, this is a way to consume it in its whole form, rather than processed which removes all the nutrition. Wheatberries also go by the name "raw wheat" or "winter wheat" at the health food store and can be bought in bulk inexpensively.

Cranberry-Wheatberry Salad

1 cup wheatberries (whole-wheat grains)
½ cup dried cranberries
1 T. extra-virgin olive oil
¼ cup oil-cured olives, pitted and chopped
    (optional)
Juice of one orange with pulp
Juice of one lemon
Salt to taste

Place the wheatberries in a pot with four cups of cold water. Bring to boil, cover, reduce heat, and boil gently for about one hour until they are chewy-tender. Drain. Toss the warm wheatberries with the remaining ingredients. Allow to cool; add salt to taste. This provides four servings with only 209 calories and 4.5 grams of fat.

Susan's Simple Tip
In a hurry for a quick lunch idea? Spoon several tablespoons of this yummy Cranberry-Wheatberry Salad on top of one or two handfuls of greens.

9. Don't Diet—Ever!

After decades of dieting and searching for "the answer" I am absolutely 100% crystal clear that diets don't work—unless you want to gain weight. You know the routine. After getting off the scale and feeling disgusted with yourself, you decide you have to do *something*. A friend at the health club or grocery store tells you about the latest diet craze. She lost 20 pounds in two months by eliminating carbohydrates from her diet. *Not a good idea!*

This latest dieting trend is concerning since it places tremendous strain on the kidneys and spleen, and it actually leaches calcium from your bones due to excess protein without a healthy balance of quality carbohydrates. And it's just like all the other weight-loss diets out there. A short-term fix for a long-term problem.

As soon as you go off any restrictive diet that leaves you feeling deprived, you go back to your old ways and quickly regain the weight plus a little more. So what's a girl (or boy) to do?

We all know deep down what it takes to lose weight—some combination of exercising more and consuming fewer calories. My experience with clients has shown me that people who exercise on a regular basis (at least four to five times a week) are *rarely* overweight. Most people who come to me for help with weight loss don't exercise regularly—or at all. The exception to this occurs when we hit the middle range of life. Especially women seem to gain weight as our hormones shift, usually 10 to 15 pounds about the time we turn 40.

One theory behind this is that the body needs the extra weight as we go into premenopause since fat cells contain more estrogen. It makes sense that this is nature's way of protecting our bones from osteoporosis. This explanation seemed perfectly logical to me—until I hit 40 and gained 15 pounds in three months. This was *after* I had improved my diet. Even more discouraging, I had been running 20-25 miles a week for 22 years. Clearly my metabolism changed and no matter how much additional exercise I did, my weight wouldn't budge.

The gift in all this was that I had to get REAL about making another shift in improving my food choices. As mentioned in #1 in this chapter, Healing Your Relationship With Food, nutrition improvements work best in stages. I was making fairly healthy choices prior to age 40 and always justified the potato chips by buying the ones cooked in olive oil—but they were still high in empty calories, offering little nutrition. I knew dieting wasn't the answer and was paranoid about feeling deprived due to my twisted history with food (see future memoir for details).

Instead, I started to write down exactly what I was eating to increase my awareness—without judgment, optimally. What I discovered is that I was less likely to eat junk food if I had to write it down in my daily planner. I re-focused on making sure I included seven fruits and veggies daily and started visualizing how it would feel to get back into my smaller jeans that had been abandoned two years previously. I did really well during the week, and not quite as well on the weekends, but finally released the excess weight. Most of it.

The exciting part was being able to make healthier choices *without feeling deprived.* I now usually substitute nuts for potato chips when the salt craving hits, and still have a small amount of good chocolate on many days. I found that when a delectable piece of chocolate is savored (without guilt and without distractions like TV), sweet cravings are satisfied with less of the treat. And when your body is no longer assaulted by white sugar regularly, fruit tastes deliciously sweet and will usually satisfy that craving. If this sounds like a foreign language, refocus on practicing acceptance of your body (#21). Perhaps the following tip (#10) will help you feel more "in control" in order to heighten your awareness as a first step.

10. Consider the Free Food Concept

I am not in favor of obsessing over food, but in the past I found counting calories helpful for increasing awareness when trying to release some extra weight. For the most part, total calories consumed minus calories expended through exercise and daily living determine whether you gain weight, release it, or stay the same.

Notice I didn't say "lose" weight. Psychologically, I wonder if we think we need to find something we've lost, so I avoid that word. After realizing I needed to further improve my eating habits due to mid-life weight gain, I invented the concept of "free food." This idea grew from making healthy choices and planning ahead for those times when my resolve to eat healthier is tested. Here's how it works:

When counting calories, there are certain foods I don't count at all due to such incredibly low calorie content and the fact that they're so good for us. They include the following: greens, carrots, celery, broccoli, green and red peppers, onion, garlic and snow peas.

These foods are "free" as long as you don't add anything like salad dressing, oils or additional calories. Not only are you managing total caloric intake with this little tool, but you're encouraging yourself to eat more vegetables— always a good thing. I no longer find it necessary to count calories; if you tend to obsess about food by doing so, focus on other tips and let this one go. But continue to eat more veggies.

11. *Plan Ahead*

What has made McDonald's and other fast food restaurants so successful? They're fast and easy. Okay, I admit it—sometimes the french fries taste great, too. But their biggest appeal is convenience. Our culture is obsessed with time; we're willing to sacrifice our health as long as we can "take back" an extra 15 minutes a day. However, even that extra 15 minutes may be an illusion. Consider how long it takes you to poll your family for their orders, get in the car and drive (in rush hour traffic, perhaps?) to your local fast food joint, sit in line while ordering and waiting for your food, drive back home and round up the troops to eat dinner.

Now consider having a few basics on hand in your fridge, pantry and freezer. This allows you to prepare dinner in the same amount of time it takes to poison yourself and your family with "fast food." There was actually a study done proving it takes no more time to create a healthy and tasty meal than it does to gather everyone's order and drive back and forth to retrieve the fast food. Amy Decision, author of *The Tightwad Gazette*, created "the pantry principle" which validates the study results. Keep certain basics—which you stock up on when they're on sale—in your pantry and freezer; this allows you to create dinner with whatever you have on hand at the moment.

In addition to the health benefits, it's also a great way to save money. We just made plans to take our whole family on a vacation and part of the way we're paying for it is by "living off the land" for two months. I peruse our available choices and create dinner from those plus the fresh produce I keep on hand. Here's an example: I sautéed carrots, celery, pepper, onion, garlic, and mushrooms for a few minutes while reheating some brown rice I had left over in the fridge. When the veggies were done, I added the brown rice along with one leftover salmon steak (broken up) that was grilled the night before and voila— dinner! The list that follows is what I like to have on hand for the pantry principle to work:

Pantry

Brown rice, wild rice, couscous, olive oil, peanut oil (for stir-frying), whole buckwheat, barley, steel-cut oats, quality marinara sauce in a jar, chicken broth, beans, split peas. Whole-grain flours and flax seeds should be stored in the fridge or freezer as they will go rancid fairly quickly.

Refrigerator

Eggs (best from a local farm, if possible), greens, broccoli, milk (raw if possible), whole plain yogurt, nuts, flax seeds.

Freezer

Whole chickens, skinless/boneless chicken breasts, ground turkey, steaks and hamburger (buffalo or beef), leftover soups, homemade chicken broth and vegetable broth, frozen juices, berries, butter, homemade pesto, and chilies from the summer's farmer's market. All of these are best when organic, especially animal protein. The freezer is a great way to take advantage of sales and will pay for itself quickly.

Produce to Keep On Hand ·

Always: garlic, onion, celery, carrots, potatoes, peppers, mushrooms, lettuce (anything but iceberg)

Often: leeks, snow peas, shallots, bok choy, cilantro, kale or other greens.

Susan's Simple Tip

Make a big pot of beans and a big pot of brown rice at the beginning of each week. They keep well in the fridge, and when you combine both with veggies you have on hand and the appropriate spices, it's the perfect side dish or entree. Example: add a can of Italian-spiced tomatoes with some oregano and basil to serve with a pasta dish or grilled fish.

12. Reduce White Flour

Do you believe you don't consume much white/refined flour? Consider the following before skipping this section: when did you last buy or eat boxed macaroni and cheese, crackers, pasta, cereal, store-bought cookies, bakery products, bread, bagels or English muffins? See what I mean? This is tricky and it takes considerable attention to significantly reduce this nutrient-depleted food. Read all food labels and put those boxes back if they don't have "whole" in front of the wheat or other grain used in them. If this sounds limiting, check out some new grain choices in #17.

Whole (unrefined) grains are healthier alternatives to refined products and more tasty. When grains are refined, as in white rice and white flour products, the nutrient-packed bran (outer layer) and germ are removed. Fortification by manufacturers replaces some B vitamins, but they're synthetic and not easily assimilated. Whenever a food has to be "fortified," due to the manufacturing process which removes some of the nutrition, leave it on the shelf.

Milling grains into flour greatly increases their tendency to disturb blood-sugar levels and insulin secretion, making them more fattening. According to Donald Yance, author of *Herbal Medicine, Healing and Cancer*, much proof exists to indicate that excessive use of processed flours and white sugars play a significant role in creating cancer and many other life-threatening diseases.

Susan's Simple Tip
Donald Yance has influenced my views and
convictions about healing greatly. He can talk
circles around many highly-educated oncologists,
yet retain the peaceful and open heart he
learned from the Franciscan monks many years
ago. Not to mention his affinity with jazz. I
know of no other herbalist with a larger library
of scientific studies and eclectic reference
books related to the efficacy of herbal medicine.
To learn more about his healing philosophy,
which I share, I invite you to visit:
NaturaHealthProducts.com

By comparison, whole grains are nutritional power-
houses, full of B vitamins, fiber, magnesium, vitamin E,
and selenium—which has been proven to reduce your
risk of cancer. Studies indicate that one to three servings
each day can cut your risk of heart disease, diabetes and
other chronic diseases. They are also a great source of
complex carbohydrates that your body needs for energy.
When shopping for cereals, breads, or other whole-grain
products, don't judge a product by color alone. Be sure
the label lists "whole grain" or "whole-wheat flour" as the
first ingredient.

Susan's Simple Tip

After taste-testing many whole-grain crackers which offered a culinary experience similar to cardboard, I discovered Ak-Mak Cracker Bread. It comes in large sheets which are easily broken into crackers and has a short list of real food ingredients. RyeKrisps and the delicious Mary's Gone Crackers are great alternatives for those avoiding wheat. Any "alternatives" I suggest aren't just "ok"—they're mahvelous, dahling.

13. Be Completely Present with Your Food

When you savor and enjoy each and every bite of food *without guilt* you will be satisfied with less—a lot less. I had a lesson years ago as I was eating alone, an unusual experience. I love the culinary delight of dining with my family, but alone, I was able to concentrate fully on how much I was enjoying every bite. My dinner consisted of six slices of toasted whole-grain baguette with brushetta (diced tomatoes, minced garlic, and fresh basil with olive oil) on top. The crowning glory was freshly grated parmesan cheese. I also had a few slices of yellow and red pepper, and a couple small pieces of delicious chocolate for dessert.

Rather than reading while eating this meal, I put my book down and savored every single bite. It was more delicious than ever and I realized that I'm often doing something else while eating—reading, talking with a friend, visiting with family, or popping up to get a forgotten item from the kitchen. Too many people eat while watching TV, which is even more distracting. If you're attention is not focused on how delicious the food is, it takes a lot more to fill you up. I love good food and am learning more all the time about how healthy, nutritious food can also taste fabulous—like the brushetta. I savored every bite, often closing my eyes to intensify the taste, and taking a deep breath after swallowing to further savor the synergy of flavors.

To some degree, this can be done while eating with others, too. Conversation will be a part of most meals you share with others, and I believe heartily in having family meal times many times a week to nurture those relationships. But having some silence as part of every meal is rather refreshing and allows us to focus solely on the food. Try it for one bite. If you enjoy it, try it for several bites. Soon you'll be loving and appreciating your food more, and eating less.

Savoring your food is especially important if you're choosing to eat potato chips or chocolate or some other "treat." If you're going to eat it, enjoy it completely and observe how little it takes to feel satisfied. In fact, the more you focus on being completely present with your food, the more you will prefer healthy food to junk food. Your body is ultimately wise and will usually choose nutritious food when given a choice. This has been demonstrated in Africa where starving children consistently choose rice gruel over sweets.

14. Flax, Flax, and More Flax

Most of us in the West are deficient in essential fatty acids (EFA's). These are otherwise known as omega-3's and omega-6's; it's the omega-3's which are especially lacking in our diet. They are found in salmon, mackerel, sardines, hemp seeds, purslane (it's a green), soybeans, walnuts, and...flax. However, if you buy farmed salmon rather than wild, it probably doesn't have the EFA's unless the salmon farmer makes sure the fish get that in their diet. My understanding is that the eggs that have omega-3's added are no better; look for eggs of chickens allowed to graze "free range."

But one of the simplest ways to incorporate more EFA's into your diet is by adding flax seeds. Flax seed oil is available at the market, but I don't recommend it. It contains no fiber, goes rancid very quickly and lacks the protective lignins found in the ground seeds. It's also a lot more expensive. I suggest keeping flax seeds in the refrigerator (up to 30 days) as they also can become rancid, especially after you grind them. The ground seeds are great for added fiber and help balance hormones by supplying your body with those omega-3's. A coffee-grinder works perfectly; use one to two tablespoons a day.

Flax seeds are safe for virtually everyone (including women who are pregnant or breastfeeding), with the possible exception of those with inflammatory bowel disease since they may have a mild laxative effect. Try sprinkling them over cereals, soups, salads, and rice. They can also be baked into muffins or bread. In fact, Susun Weed, author of many wonderful herb books, says they're even more beneficial when heated in our own ovens. Two recipes follow which are simple ways to include ground flax seeds in your diet.

Oatmeal with Flaxseeds

⅔ cup oats
1½ cup water
2 T. ground raw flaxseeds
2-4 T. blueberries (ok to nuke briefly if frozen)
½ cup organic (preferably raw) cow's milk
2 t. Honey

Boil water, stir in oats and return to boil. Reduce heat to medium low. Cook uncovered for 5 minutes, stirring occasionally. Remove from heat and let stand a few minutes. Stir in ground flaxseeds, plain and whole yogurt, blueberries, and honey. Top with sliced banana if desired.

Susan's Simple Tip

Grind up a cup or more of flax seeds and store in an airtight glass container inside the refrigerator. This makes them easy to add to your smoothie or salad.

Malted Cinnamon Crunch

1 cup flaxseeds, ground in coffee grinder
⅓ cup barley malt
2-3 t. ground cinnamon

Preheat oven to 350° F. Grind the flaxseeds in an electric coffee grinder one-third cup at a time. Place the ground seeds in a bowl. Pour the malt into a small saucepan and bring to a boil. Allow to boil for one minute while stirring. Pour the hot malt over the ground seeds and add the cinnamon. Stir until the malt coats the seeds evenly. Spread this mixture on a cookie sheet sprayed with olive oil and bake 10 minutes. Cool on wax paper and store in an airtight container. This provides a serving of plant estrogen in every bite. You can also use it instead of sugar on hot cereal.

15. Onions, Garlic, and Ginger— The Three Musketeers Fighting for Your Immune System

As an herbalist it's common to see clients with chronic colds, flu, ear infections, or sinus congestion. These are pretty simple to manage with herbs, as our ancestors have for centuries. But if you're sick more than once or twice a year, your body is asking for a change. All of us have certain body systems or organs that are more susceptible to disease and imbalance. For some it's gastrointestinal problems; for others, the sinus cavities. Some people get so far out of balance, their immune systems attack themselves, resulting in autoimmune disorders.

The Chinese believe that our first medicine needs to be food and I couldn't agree more. This is one of the simplest ways to increase your body's ability to fight off a bacteria or virus. The bonus is it's free medicine because we all need to eat anyway. When you start eating whole foods rather than fast-food burgers and meals out of a box filled with chemicals, it will also decrease your food bill significantly. And now that you have all these simple tips and recipes at your fingertips, plus the Timesavers listed in Chapter Seven, you will learn to eat healthier without stressing about it.

Trust me, after the adrenaline-pumping days of most Americans, coming home to the basics stocked in your own kitchen to prepare a tasty and wholesome meal for your family can be a pleasure for you and a gift of love for your family. But are you too tired to stand at the stove? Try this:

breathe deeply through your nose and lift tall through the crown of your head as you lift the sole of one foot to the calf of your opposite leg. You're in "tree pose" which will take the weight off one leg at a time for a bit of rest; it also helps you breathe, lift up tall and improve your balance while you remember—trees sway in the wind sometimes.

When I see chronic illnesses in my clients I almost always recommend including onions, garlic, and ginger in their daily diet. These three foods have been shown to increase a healthy immune response. They will not only protect you from the common cold, but will decrease your risk of developing cancer, heart disease, and diabetes.

If anything is good for you and your health, it's garlic. It helps balance cholesterol and blood pressure, decrease excess clotting in the blood, and strengthen the immune

My Second Husband's Template For a Simple Italian Meal

Sautee fresh minced garlic (plus onion, if desired) in olive oil for a couple minutes before adding vegetables and one of the following for protein: beans, shrimp, clams, beef, tempeh, chicken. Complete your meal with a red marinara sauce or white clam sauce plus lots of fresh herbs to protect you from cancer. Mangiare! Mangiare! (Eat! Eat! In Italian)

I give culinary thanks for this to my second husband, Rusty—a hot Italiano.

system as a potent antibiotic without the side effects. Combined with onions and ginger on a daily basis, it will help you ward off colds, flus, and sinus infections after just one season of daily use.

I start many meals with olive oil, garlic, and onion since from there you can get creative with a variety of vegetables, fermented soy products, and hormone-free meats and poultry. The medicinal properties of garlic are greater if it's raw. Try using some to flavor the dish, then adding some fresh, uncooked garlic just before serving. I'm including a couple of recipes here to get you started on this thrilling threesome of medicinal plants.

Ginger-Carrot Soup

3 cups chopped carrots
1 medium chopped potato
8 cups vegetable stock (homemade or canned
    without additives)
1 medium chopped onion
2 t. olive oil
2-3 T. finely chopped fresh ginger root (easily
    obtained at any market)
salt to taste
dash of nutmeg
chopped fresh parsley or cilantro (optional)

Dice the carrots and potato in your food processor and combine with the vegetable stock in a soup pot.

Ginger-Carrot Soup (continued)

I leave the skins on for extra fiber and nutrients. Bring to a boil, cover, reduce heat, and boil gently until the veggies are tender, about 10-15 minutes. Meanwhile, chop the onion, heat the oil in a skillet and add the onion and ginger, sautéing and stirring a few times until onion is translucent. Remove from heat.

When carrots and potato are tender, add the onion and ginger to the pot and cook together for 5 minutes. Add salt to taste and flavor with nutmeg. Serve plain or garnish with chopped parsley or cilantro. I love the spiciness of cilantro and it's a great protector from cancer. Serve with a loaf of hearty peasant bread (darker and whole grain) and olive oil or butter—delicious and nutritious!

Note: Many caution wisely not to take garlic simultaneously with a pharmaceutical blood thinner like Coumadin—which you can cut down on or eventually eliminate with the help of garlic—this along with the guidance of a wise health care practitioner and regular blood tests.

Lemon Leeks

4 leeks, chopped
1 onion, chopped
2 parsnips, chopped (optional)
1 carrot, chopped
1 tomato, chopped
Juice of ½-1 lemon
White wine (optional)
Chopped parsley (optional)
Optional fresh or dried herbs (marjoram, rosemary,
    thyme, sage)

Sauté the leeks, onion, parsnips, and carrot in one tsp. olive oil on medium low heat. Add a little water and white wine if desired. Cover and simmer until tender, about 10-15 minutes. Add chopped parsley, tomato, salt, pepper, any fresh or dried herbs you like, and the fresh lemon juice. Simmer a few more minutes. There should be a little sauce created by the liquids.

This is a variation of a Sephardic Jewish dish and makes a delicious and comforting meal or side dish. Feel free to add fresh, minced ginger for a little more spice and one more immune booster!

16. Why Buy Organic?

Years ago, I scoffed at organic produce and the whole idea of toxins from our environment ending up in our bodies, but not any longer. After witnessing many health imbalances in my clients and discovering what may be best for their healing, I'm convinced that what we put into our physical "covering" makes a difference. Given the fact that we, along with trees and plants, are bombarded daily with millions of tons of pollutants in the water, air and soil, we need all the help we can get. Organic farms tend to be smaller in size, resulting in a higher cost per acre of food, but if you're reducing your consumption of junk food, that pricey poison alone can make up the difference in cost. Another option that is healthy for all of us is becoming a member of a farm coop. One fine example of this type of community farming is *HappyHeartFarmCSA.com*.

Generally speaking, certified organic food has not been treated with synthetic pesticides or herbicides—though in some instances, it will be sprayed with preservatives after picking for shipment. For food to be certified organic, the use of genetically modified ingredients is also prohibited, as is the use of biosolids, processed sewage sludge and irradiation.

Due to consumer demand, the USDA is becoming stricter in requirements for food that is certified organic. Cattle and poultry referred to as "free-range" are required to have access to pasture and be free from antibiotic and growth-hormone use. Organic foods are increasingly popular; sales were estimated at $7.76 billion worldwide in

2000 and have been growing 20 percent annually. The reasons I support organically-grown food are two-fold: better health for you, and to regain planet Earth's health.

After reading the paragraph above, is there any doubt organic foods are better for us? Granted, organic farmers leave their tractors running next to the crops occasionally, but to eliminate all those added pesticides, growth hormones, and sludge residue from our food supply *has* to be better for us. If you ever drive through rural areas, notice the difference in how you feel driving past a feedlot and passing cattle contentedly grazing in a pasture. It's palpable.

Regarding the Earth's sustenance, farming has become big business. In order to compete, most farmers have become convinced that millions of dollars have to be spent on pesticides, herbicides and synthetic fertilizers. Ironically, many of these salt-of-the-Earth folks are being bought out by developers and big business; they feel they have no choice but to sell due to the rising costs and flat commodity prices. But those who remain and are saving the soil through good farming practices are making a living at it while returning to the old-fashioned ways of using natural fertilizers and using certain insects (ladybugs, for example) to eat other insects that threaten crops.

Native Americans believe none of us actually "owns" land, but are stewards of the Earth instead. When you support sustainable farming with your purchase of organic foods it reaffirms your connection to the Earth and makes you a caring steward for future generations. For a source of pesticide-free produce, search online for a farmer's market close to you.

Susan's Simple Tip
If you live in an area without access to organic
produce, use a vegetable scrubber with soap
and water to thoroughly scrub your produce.
Don't reduce your consumption of fruits and
vegetables simply because of pesticide concerns.
I believe that *worrying* about not eating organic
food is more damaging than the chemicals on
commercial produce. Be grateful for your food
and it will nourish you.

#17. Broaden Your Use of Grains

I see a number of clients with food allergies, often due to eating the "same ol' thing" too often for years. Once you break away from white flour, it's easy to think only of whole wheat. Delicious and nutritious as it can be, there are a growing number of people in this country suffering from celiac spru, due in part to over-reliance on wheat, especially the heavily-processed flours.

Research Tip: If you have been diagnosed with celiac disease or are questioning a wheat or gluten sensitivity, the best in the business is a wonderful friend and client of mine who has celiac disease, Gina Mohr-Callahan. Her email is *AForkIntheRoad@msn.com*. She and her immunologist husband, Gerry, are both chefs and are a brilliant support option for those who struggle with these challenging issues. For more information on celiac disease, do a search with that term on *WestonAPrice.org*.

There are many other grains we can enjoy besides wheat; we just need to know what they are and how to work with them. Here are a few easily obtainable grains that offer a wide array of healing nutrients:

Buckwheat—a great alternative for those dealing with a wheat allergy or celiac spru since it contains no gluten. You can purchase it as soba—Japanese noodles—at your local Asian food market or health food store. However, if you're wheat-sensitive, read the ingredients carefully since many soba noodles on the market are combined with wheat flour. It's also a staple in Russia and Eastern Europe, where it's commonly eaten as kasha (roasted, cracked seeds). It has a robust, earthy taste.

There are several kasha breakfast cereals available at most markets. However, I encourage you to avoid cold cereals; the natural oils become very similar to hydrogenated oils when heated for extrusion purposes. A warm breakfast or a smoothie, depending on the season, is far superior for nutrition and flavor. Buckwheat flour works well as a substitute for white/wheat flour for pancakes and baked goods.

Quinoa (pronounced KEEN-wa)—a small, pearl-shaped grain-like seed of the Andes that is becoming popular here in the U.S. It contains no gluten and works well with sautéed vegetables and mushrooms. You can even use it to make a dessert pudding! Quinoa should be rinsed in a strainer before cooking to remove its bitter coating. It's a complete protein, so is helpful for vegetarian/vegan eaters. It does have a distinctive flavor, though, so it's best enjoyed in a baked product when combined with other gluten-free flours.

Oats—for great heart support. In the past, people with gluten intolerance have been advised to avoid oats because they have always been milled on the same equipment as wheat and were cross-contaminated with wheat. Now, however, there are several sources of clean, GF(gluten-free) oats available, including a Bob's Red Mill option as well as a Wyoming ranch family that produces only GF oats. See *GlutenFreeOats.com* for more information. If you don't have gluten concerns, steel cut oats from the health food store offer the most fiber. Regular rolled oats are a decent option, too—but certainly not in those individual packets riddled with sugar!

Wild Rice—not actually rice, but the seed of a tall aquatic grass, native to North America. Wild rice serves up twice as much protein and higher levels of B vitamins than other types of rice. It's rich, nutty flavor is great for casseroles, salads, stir-fries, and stuffing; the dark color adds visual interest to your plate, too. Read labels if you have concerns about cross-contamination with wheat or tree nuts. And be aware of the importance of maintaining the delicate ecological balance needed for sustainable harvesting of wild rice. For information on the impact on indigenous people and the Earth in regard to wild rice harvesting practices, please do a search on the blog found at *rastaseed.wordpress.com*.

Amaranth—popular in Africa and Latin America, it is especially helpful for those with elevated needs such as nursing or pregnant women, children, or those who do heavy physical work. Amaranth contains protein complexes that are more than adequate for many individuals, especially when combined with whole wheat or oats, added to dilute its intense flavor. It is a hearty addition to soups, but has a strong flavor and its texture is a little gritty.

Barley—familiar to most of us, especially in soups, barley has a sweet and salty flavor and strengthens the spleen, pancreas, gall bladder, and intestines. It is easily digested but can worsen cases of constipation if roasted. In addition to using it in soups or as a cereal, barley can be baked into a pseudo meatloaf with lentils and sunflower seeds.

Millet—known as "the queen of the grains," millet is "cooling" in nature—so helpful for those in various stages of menopause or if you just "run hot." It acts as a natural diuretic and strengthens the kidneys and stomach while sweetening the breath by retarding bacterial growth. It helps prevent miscarriage and is one of the best grains for those with Candida albicans. When roasted it can also be useful for diarrhea, vomiting, and diabetes. Often cooked with little or no salt, it can be served with onions and carrots as a side dish or included in casseroles.

Sorghum—with a flavor similar to wheat and more protein than rice this one's a favorite of those searching for a gluten-free flour. It's an ancient cereal crop, and there are several types of sorghum grown throughout the world, such as cane sorghum and sweet sorghum.

Teff—another great gluten-free grass from Africa, high in fiber, protein, and calcium. It's the main ingredient in injera bread (Ethiopian flat bread). *Woman's Day* magazine recently touted teff as one of ten perfect foods.

Coconut flour—one of the most nutritious and delicious gluten-free flours, coconut flour is excellent for baking. It's simply pulverized, unsweetened coconut which has great anti-inflammatory properties and yields baked goods with a light, slightly nutty/sweet flavor when combined with other GF flours.

For recipe ideas, check out the cookbooks listed in the Bibliography.

18. Eliminate Poison Foods

There are many forms of poison out there which are cleverly disguised as food. The foods and food ingredients that are most toxic to your body and most likely to promote cancer, diabetes, heart disease, and autoimmune disorders are as follows:

High Fructose Corn Sugar

Originally I had trans fatty acids (TFA's) as the number one poison on this list. However, after learning about the dangers of high fructose corn syrup (HFCS) and how ubiquitous it is in pre-packaged foods, I decided it merited the number one spot. You'll soon see why.

The consumption of fructose (aka corn syrup and high fructose corn syrup) has risen considerably in the general population within recent years. In 1980, the average person consumed 39 pounds of fructose and 84 pounds of sucrose. In 1994 the average person ate 83 pounds of fructose and 66 pounds of sucrose. This 149 pounds is approximately 19% of the average person's diet.

Corn syrup is much cheaper than table sugar (sucrose) and twice as sweet. It is absorbed less than half as quickly as glucose and causes only a modest rise in blood sugar. The medical community recommended it because of a low increase in glucose in the blood. Sounds good so far, especially for diabetics, right? But other physical changes were ignored. Let's look at some of these factors now:

◆ Fructose has no enzymes, vitamins, and minerals; it therefore robs the body of its micronutrient treasures.

◆ Research shows that fructose causes a general increase in both the total serum cholesterol and in the low density lipoproteins (LDL) in most people, resulting in a heightened risk of heart disease.

◆ Fructose is absorbed primarily in the jejunum and metabolized in the liver. Diarrhea can be a consequence, and get this: fructose/HFCS actually **shuts off your body's natural ability to know when you are no longer hungry**. Fructose also converts to fat more than any other sugar. This may be one of the reasons Americans continue to get fatter.

◆ Fructose/HFCS interacts with oral contraceptives and elevates insulin levels in women on birth control pills.

◆ Fructose and sorbitol are often substituted for glucose in IV (intravenous) feeding. This can have severe consequences with people with hereditary fructose intolerance, a congenital disorder affecting one in 21,000 people.

◆ Fructose inhibits copper metabolism. A deficiency in copper leads to bone fragility, anemia, defects of the connective tissue, arteries and bone, infertility, heart arrhythmias, high cholesterol levels, heart attacks, and an inability to control blood sugar levels.

Susan's Simple Tip
For more detailed information on High
Fructose Corn Syrup concerns, see
mercola.com/2002/jan/5/fructose.htm and
other web sites.

Trans-Fatty Acids

Also known as hydrogenated or partially hydrogenated
oil, these are the worst forms of fat you can consume.
During the process of hydrogenation, these oils are heated
until they create a significant fraction of an unnatural
species called trans-fatty acids, or TFA's. They can un-
balance your hormonal systems that regulate healing;
they lead to the construction of defective cell membranes,
and they encourage the development of cancer. The challenge to eliminating them is related to how ubiquitous
they are; most processed foods contain these dangerous
fats and somehow the FDA still permits their presence in
the manufacturing process. I hope that accumulating
medical evidence about the harmfulness of hydrogenated
oils will eventually force them to be eliminated from
prepared food products.

The only way to protect yourself from TFA's is by
reading the labels of every food you buy. You'll find hydrogenated oil listed on the labels of most crackers, snack
foods, baked goods, spreads, cookies, cereal, ice cream, as
well as other pre-packaged food. Ingredients are listed by

the quantity of each item, so the higher up on the list of ingredients, the greater the amount of TFA's.

Margarine is just one example of a food containing TFA's, and even if it says there aren't any, be aware that these products can contain up to one-half percent TFA's without having to include it on the label. Notice they say 0 grams *per serving*. If it's a choice between butter and margarine, always choose butter.

Cholesterol is the featured "bad guy" in mainstream nutrition, but the TFA's are much worse for you than cholesterol. The dangers of high cholesterol are over-blown by the medical community and the media. In fact, there is a high correlation between fertility problems and low cholesterol. See #83 to learn more about the "Cholesterol Crock."

Soda

Whether diet or regular, soda is a poison food due to the big load of artificial food colors and sulphites. In addition, one can of regular soda has 10 teaspoons of sugar, 150 calories and 30 to 55 mg of caffeine. Since the chemicals in aspartame (NutriSweet) and saccharin have been proven to cause cancer in laboratory animals (disgusting on its own), you may be making a worse choice with diet soda than the excess sugar in regular. Splenda's no better; don't be a guinea pig for these new artificial sweeteners that come out constantly.

Have your kids ever done the test at school where they drop a penny into a can of coke, learning the coke dissolves it completely? Why would we want to put that acid-on-steroids into our stomachs? Fruit juices with added water are a reasonable substitute in the beginning, but they still contain a lot of sugar.

Choose water and herbal teas instead; green tea is especially beneficial since it contains antioxidants. If you're really hooked on sodas, back off gradually as the caffeine withdrawal can cause nasty headaches. Sparkling mineral water with lemon or lime added is a reasonable substitute for other carbonated beverages.

Susan's Simple Tip

Caffeine Comparison—Coffee has 125-185 mg per cup, Black Tea, 25-55 mg per cup, and Green Tea contains four to 32 mg per cup. My preference is to drink two to three cups of weak black tea, and one to three cups of green tea; not because that's the healthiest balance—it's just what I like. I came across a cool web site on tea while doing my research. Check it out: *teatimeworldwide.com*.

Fast Food

The most effective way to eliminate fast food is to ask your server for the nutritional information on each item you've been eating; the information can be really scary. For example, if you're trying to release extra weight, you'll be astounded at the calories in fast foods. Another concern is the oils they use for frying. Most of them are on the "bad" list of fats (#19), and often are in use so long, their stability is further decreased. If you can't quit cold-turkey, at least consider the Mexican burrito chains or Asian food chains. Their choices are often superior to burgers and fries, but ask that any MSG be left out.

And remember that you rarely save time with fast food. If you learn to plan ahead, it takes less time to eat wholesome foods that you feel good about eating. And when you do enjoy dining out, ask your server what type of oil they use to cook with, and whether any of their meats are hormone-free and antibiotic-free. Wild game is often a healthier choice.

Chemicals

It sounds simple to not eat chemicals, doesn't it? Start reading those ingredient labels and you'll soon learn how many synthetic dyes, flavorings, and colorings are in our "food." I have two general rules to help you find your way through this maze: the longer the ingredient list is, the more likely you'll find chemicals, and if you can't pronounce it, don't eat it. Even when shopping at a health food store, read the labels. Just because these stores offer healthier choices doesn't mean everything they sell is good for you.

Some of the biggest culprits for containing chemicals in our food are poultry, meat, and dairy products. It is a little more expensive to buy these products without growth hormones and antibiotics, but those chemicals are passed on to us when we eat them. Ever wonder why young girls are menstruating at a much earlier age than in the past? It's been suggested it's partly due to ingesting growth hormones in animal products. And with the overuse of antibiotics we already take, we don't need to add more of them to challenge our immune systems. Many Americans consume at least twice as much animal protein as needed; cut back on the quantity, and focus on the quality of your food to stay within your budget.

Susan's Simple Tip
Don't be fooled by a listing of "partially hydrogenated coconut oil," since no matter how healthy the oil is initially, the hydrogenation process greatly damages it with high heat.

19. Tips for Travelers

Traveling brings special challenges for making healthy food choices. Airline food is nearly non-existent. On the rare occasions when a meal is available during your flight, it's most likely to be overpriced and under nourishing. When traveling or commuting to work, take along any of the following for survival foods:

> nuts and seeds
> dried fruit
> fresh fruit and vegetables
> real fruit juices
> watered down soups, in a thermos
> herbal tea bags (chamomille will help you relax)
> whole-grain breads and crackers
> quality granola from the health food store

Snacks can be carried in small plastic bags or containers, Mason jars, etc. Canvas carrying bags with a shoulder strap, lined with washable, water-resistant fabric or plastic, can be purchased at discount stores or health food stores. Sometimes leftovers can be used, or quick foods prepared in the morning.

Stopping at a roadside restaurant is a welcome break, but the menu is often less than optimal. If you have munched on good snacks along the way, you won't feel the need to order something you may regret later. Most roadside restaurants have clear soups, salad bars (choose wisely) and eggs. Regarding eggs, it's best to cook them with the yolk whole (soft-boiled and hard-boiled) due to oxidation, but don't be paranoid—eggs in any form are a healthier choice than many restaurant options. Another alternative is a health food store with a cafe in it for some nice alternatives.

See Appendix D for a list of my Favorite Foods— yummy!

Chapter Two

Exercise for the
Rest of Us

"Lack of activity destroys the good condition
of every human being, while movement and methodical
physical exercise save it and preserve it."

Plato

Cindy, a 44-year-old mother of three busy teenagers, came to see me about hormone fluctuations that started in her late thirties. Her irritability, frequent bloating and weepiness had lessened while she was on HRT (hormone replacement therapy), but after the Women's Health Initiative was stopped in 2002 due to concerns regarding an increase in both heart disease and breast cancer for those on HRT, Cindy didn't want to take the chance of having her family's history of heart disease catch up with her. Like many women, she was advised to quit HRT abruptly, rather than gradually decreasing her dosage while using herbal remedies and good common sense to help with her transition.

Shortly after turning 40, Cindy gained 18 pounds which seemed impervious to her low-fat diet. This didn't surprise me, and I felt confident that increasing the quality fat in Cindy's diet would reduce her sugar cravings and help her release at least some of those extra pounds. Adding a consistent exercise program would not only speed her return to a height-appropriate weight, but also help protect her from heart disease, increase her energy level and help balance her emotions. Cindy was reluctant since she already felt pushed for time and was embarrassed to be seen in a group exercise class; but she was willing to start with a five minute daily walk—outside, weather permitting. At first she scoffed at whether five minutes could make a difference, but I asked her to try it for a month.

When we met just four weeks later, she reported being a consistent walker five to six days a week, and when, on several occasions, it felt like an especially beautiful day, she stretched her walk to 10 or 15 minutes. And she actually enjoyed it! Being outside helped her focus on her breath and leave her worries behind for a short time; she said her energy level had risen from a four to a six on a one-to-ten scale. Though feeling mildly discouraged at "only" dropping three pounds in a month, she decided it was worthwhile enough to commit to 15 minutes a day for the next month.

She was still eating fast food and junk food frequently, but noticed that her cravings for sugar and junk food were less on the days following a day of mostly healthy choices, including organic butter, olive oil, a few nuts and perhaps some guacamole with whole-grain chips. After another four weeks of doing a bit better with traditional whole foods and finding 15 minutes to walk five or six days a week, Cindy's skin started to clear, her energy level rose to an eight and a half and she released another five pounds.

Fast and glamorous? No. But it was a great start to a new, and hopefully lifelong, way of living. Her blood pressure even dropped several points and she now felt committed to increasing her walks to 30 minutes and adding a weekly yoga class for strength development and stress relief. Within four months, Cindy had released 16 of the extra 18 pounds, reported an energy level of 10, and most importantly, her self-esteem was higher. She attributed this to making healthier choices and feeling less irritable around her family.

It can happen for you, too. Read on.

20. Accept Your Body—As Is

Exercise is critical if you want to be healthy, live longer, and maintain a reasonable weight. When I work with new clients concerned about their weight, regular exercise is the single thing that makes the greatest difference. If you want to release excess weight, it is absolutely imperative to move your body. However, if you start an exercise program while judging your body harshly, it will be a miracle if you stick with it. You can't do something loving and supportive of yourself, like exercising regularly, if you hate your body. The ironic thing is that the more you practice acceptance of your body's appearance and how it functions, the more you'll be able to improve it through exercise.

Try this form of meditation while learning to accept your body in its current state. While sitting quietly with your eyes closed, think or say to yourself "I love and appreciate my beautiful body." Then mentally list each and every body part you are striving to love and appreciate. "I love and appreciate my beautiful face, I love and appreciate my beautiful arms, I love and appreciate my beautiful chest." When you come to the parts of your body you've been most critical of, say the sentence twice, and say it slower. It sounds cheesy, but fake it until you begin to believe it. This alone will change how you feel about your body over a period of several weeks, or maybe months if you've been particularly harsh with yourself. If quiet time sounds like a fantasy, this form of meditation can be done while driving—with your eyes open. While this was a big issue for me, my favorite spot was in the sauna after a workout with my eyes closed.

Journaling (#63) is another great way to make peace with your body. You may want to have a separate journal (or a 49 cent spiral notebook) just for this purpose. Write about the ways you have abused your body and your self. This may not be fun, but it is very healing to become aware of judgments made by yourself and others. With this type of writing it's important not to self-edit as you go; don't worry about grammar, misspellings or stupid phrases. Look at it as a mind-dump to prevent you from internalizing negative thoughts that affect your body. One of my clients burns pages she has written to insure she doesn't beat up on herself even more by re-reading.

After working out the past negative judgments of yourself and others, try writing down all the things you appreciate about your body. Whether you judge how it looks or how it functions, this is a great exercise for self-healing. If you're seriously overweight, appreciate your beautiful skin, a nice smile, a sparkle in your eyes, or mischief in your soul. And if you haven't had heart issues yet, that is clearly something to be grateful for; don't wait for a heart attack to make changes.

Next, make amends to your body for all the cruel things you've said and thought about it. Making amends doesn't just mean saying your sorry; it's a vow to do better in the future. Do that—please. Because even if you never drop a pound, self-acceptance can improve your health and be the greatest gift you've ever received.

If you're vowing to do better in the future with self care than you have previously, consider the following definition of forgiveness:

Forgiveness = letting go of all hope for a different past

21. Getting Started

Beginning is the hardest part for most of us. If you've become a couch potato over the years, or have never enjoyed sports or exercise of any type, getting started is definitely your biggest hurdle. How to hoist that sedentary, perhaps overweight body off the sofa, over the hurdle, and out the door? Do it one foot at a time. I want you to start s-l-o-w-l-y.

If you're out of shape, you may feel temporarily motivated by a New Year's resolution, by an inconsiderate remark from someone you've now removed from your Blackberry, or by taking a look in the mirror at the beginning of swimsuit season. Once this happens, you probably resolve to do *something* about it and throw yourself into whatever the latest craze is on TV. STOP!

Before starting any exercise program, do an assessment of what your body is actually able to do. That may include a trip to your doctor's office for a stress test, or perhaps just a self-assessment of what's working and what feels stiff or unwilling to move. If the only exercise you've had lately is picking up the television remote, check with your health care practitioner first. If you are literally so large it's difficult to get off the sofa, you can always start with some isometric exercises to build a little muscle.

Once you know your starting point, consider what might actually be fun, or at least enjoyable. What did you do as a kid that you thought was fun? Fly a kite, play soccer, kick a can around the block, run in a field with your dog—all of these are still options. I believe everyone has some form of physical activity that is fun for them, and if you enjoy it, you're more likely to stick with it. Don't limit yourself to the same thing every day; mix it up to keep your interest alive.

If you're debating about what form of exercise to try and are coming up with zero, get a comfortable pair of appropriate shoes and start walking (#22). Most of us can get outside for a walk at least four to five days a week. If the weather interferes, try walking indoors at your local shopping mall. If you live in Alaska where snow and ice are the norm, get the dog sled or snowshoes dusted off, and dress in layers since you'll heat up quickly.

Ask a friend to join you if that will increase your dedication to sticking with it. Too embarrassed to be seen in public? There are plenty of exercise videos, but be sure to start with one geared for beginners. And if this is the toughest area for you to simplify, think of a reward for yourself that doesn't involve a trip to McDonalds! My favorite "treat" is putting my feet up for 15 minutes with a good novel.

22. Walking

An underrated form of exercise, walking will burn almost as many calories per mile as running, but with less chance of injury. It does take a bit more time; I used to use that as an excuse, too. Then I injured my piraformis muscle (located at the base of the bum), forcing me to quit running after 22 years. At 42 and with legs I describe as strong tree trunks rather than those of a gazelle, it was a gift, because my body was ready for a gentler approach. That happened over eight years ago and I haven't missed running. For a while I used a reclining bike at the health club three times a week because I was afraid I'd gain weight if I only walked. Not so. I now walk a brisk 45 to 60 minute loop on most days, but it feels more like a present-moment meditation than exercise. I gratefully soak up vitamin D from the sun, and delight in being part of the change of seasons, rather than just an observer.

If your goal is moving your body daily, you'll likely get it in five to six days a week. Many people sabotage themselves by aiming for three to four days a week since that is what is recommended for a minimal sense of fitness; but in our busy culture, plans change frequently. Consider getting your workout first thing in the morning to minimize those inevitable interferences. If walking alone, vary your route occasionally so you don't get bored. Focus on how many items of beauty you can find along the way. Simple things like bulbs coming up in the spring or leaves turning color in the fall will warm your heart and make you smile. Even on days when you're tempted to hit the snooze button, I guarantee you'll be glad you went for a walk once you get outside and moving.

Regarding equipment, there is no need for fancy Reeboks at $100 a pair. You can often find good prices on comfortable walking shoes at Target or other discount stores. When you find some you especially like, stock up with an extra pair. When it's wet or snowy outside, you can put on a pair of hiking boots or those combination sneaker/boots. Cotton socks absorb the sweat and are available in a heavier weight for winter warmth. Walking year around is a special treat and you'll soon learn how to layer your clothing based on the temperature. Sunglasses are often desirable in the summer (though they do block Vitamin D absorption) and sometimes a hat feels right, especially on bad hair days. If you're committed to doing your part for neighborhood clean-up, you may want to carry a small plastic bag for picking up trash.

Are you significantly out of shape, recuperating from an illness, or telling yourself you don't have time? Start with just five to ten minutes a day. Nearly everyone can make time for that, and once you get started, you'll build the necessary strength and stamina for longer walks. Most people enjoy walking, but if you really hate it, find something else that's fun. Life is too short to grit your teeth while exercising.

23. Going That Extra Foot

I know if I suggest a mile you won't read this. What I'm referring to is parking a little further away from the grocery store, taking the stairs instead of the elevator, or walking the short distance that sometimes exists between errands. Think of it as creating time alone to focus on nature all around you—even if you have to look over concrete to see the beauty. Turn on some music while vacuuming. The Beatles are great for increasing your pace and having some fun. When the music moves you to dance, do it! It will feel good, give you some additional exercise, and make you smile. At work, walk to someone's office for a chat rather than always using email. This is especially important if it's a "hot" topic since you may spout off things in an email that you would never say in person.

24. Running

I love this form of exercise, mostly because it can be done outdoors. For some, a treadmill is a better option, but I can't imagine wanting to trade the outdoors for a television. If you've never run before, start with brisk walking to build up your stamina over a two to three week period. At that point, you can start out on your walk, breaking into an easy jog after a few minutes and return to walking if you start to feel out of breath. One woman in our neighborhood has been doing a combination of running and walking for years—complete with a coffee mug in her hand! Isn't it great that there aren't any rules?

Eventually, you may want to work up to 20 or 30 minutes at whatever pace feels right. If you're trying to release some extra pounds, consider getting a heart rate monitor and asking a personal trainer for guidance. If you get more serious about running, I suggest mixing up your workouts. After running three to five days a week for a few weeks, work up to 30 minutes or more and experiment with the schedule that appears on the following page.

If you start to train more seriously, having a rest day is critical. It not only gives your body time to rest and rebuild, it gives you a nice break mentally. Otherwise, this starts to feel like a grind. Once you follow a schedule similar to the one below for a few months, you may want to experiment with "interval" days on Tuesdays and Thursdays. Intervals involve starting your run at a slow, warm-up pace; then increasing your speed significantly for one to two minutes. Go back and forth between five minutes

Mondays	30 minute run at medium pace (8-minute miles)
Tuesdays	30 minute brisk walk or 15 to 20 minutes slightly faster run (7- to 8-minute miles)
Wednesdays	30 minute run at medium pace (8-minute miles)
Thursdays	30 minute brisk walk or 15-20 minutes slightly faster run (7- to 8-minute miles)
Fridays	30 minute run at medium pace (8-minute miles)
Saturdays	60 minute run at slow pace (9- to10-minute miles)
Sundays	Rest!

at a slow-to-medium pace and one to two minutes flat-out fast. It can keep your interest and is a very good tool if you want to train for road races.

Running is not essential for good health. These recommendations are based on my personal running experience, and are offered for those who think running sounds like a fun sport. Walking or gentle jogging gives you enough of a cardiovascular workout for a healthy body. This tip provides you with an option if you like to mix things up a bit or want to train safely for a road race. If you have days when you don't feel like running, try some other form of activity; just keep moving your body on a regular basis. And, by the way, it's not a coincidence there's a book (sadly, out of print) titled *The Runners' Yoga Book* by Jean Couch. If you run, I highly recommend adding yoga, as well. But then, I recommend yoga to everyone.

25. Weight-Lifting

Though some of us aspire to having "buff" bodies, lifting weights is in no way a requirement for good health. If you walk and stretch or practice yoga regularly you will have all you need for optimal health. But if the idea of feeling strong or creating more muscle definition is appealing, please follow the guidelines below to keep your body free of injury.

◆ First check with your physician to get his or her approval; then make an appointment with a *good* personal trainer. Ask your friends who they've used or ask your trusted health care practitioner who they would recommend. A well-educated trainer will help you achieve better results faster, with minimum exposure to injury. If you have time constraints—and who doesn't?—let your trainer know that efficiency is also important.

◆ If weight lifting is foreign to you, take notes on the sheet your trainer will provide to help you remember the machines or free weights you used, the number of reps (repetitions) you did, and how many sets (groups of repetitions) you want to lift. Take your time and move slowly since this actually creates more benefit and keeps you injury-free. It also helps you maintain awareness of your breath.

◆ Listen to your body! If something creates pain, don't do it. Period. Your trainer can help you

discover what may be causing the pain, but you
will regret it if you push too hard, too fast.

◆ Stretch in between sets, or at least when you
have finished with each machine or free-weight
exercise. A trainer suggested I do this and,
as a yoga teacher, I'm embarrassed to admit
that I hadn't even thought of it. Your trainer
can guide you in an appropriate stretch for the
muscle group you just used and it makes a big
difference in muscle recovery. You have to do
something anyway for at least 45 seconds
between sets, so make the time beneficial.
Your body will thank you.

Weight lifting can be especially empowering for
women, but be careful if you're tempted to cross the line
into body-building. From a health perspective, it is too
much of a good thing, and often comes with advice to
severely restrict your diet and/or use potentially harmful
supplements. Instead, I suggest a life of balance.

26. Yoga—Or at Least, Stretching

This practice is a wonderful way to "exercise" your body, but its benefits are far more than physical. There is a stillness inside after practicing yoga. This sense of peace comes from slowing down, focusing on the breath, and listening to our bodies for feedback and instruction. I find it heightens my awareness in all things and guides me to living in the present moment.

It's my belief that everyone can benefit from yoga, even if they are bedridden. And now that Oprah has had Rodney Yee—one of my most impressive instructors—on her television show, we know it's hit the mainstream. For good reason. Yoga is not only great for developing flexibility and a calmer mind; it can be very strengthening as well. The true benefit of yoga is creating the ability to live fully, breathe deeply and accept life on life's terms.

I specialize in teaching "beginners." There's nothing more exciting than observing a middle-aged woman, decades from her last workout, who feels better after her first yoga class. Or the 62-year old guy who never thought he could practice yoga and now raves about how it is helping his cycling and golf game.

However, I'm not excited about some of the yoga offered at certain health clubs and chains—especially for beginners. It is common for instructors at *some* of them to be aerobics teachers who received a certification in yoga after only a weekend of training. If you already belong to a health club (well done) and actually use it (even better), ask about the credentials of your instructors and whether they have classes targeted for beginners, or those with special needs. In addition to several months of study before certification, I'd like to see all yoga teachers further their education on an annual basis.

If you don't belong to a health club, consider using that monthly fee for yoga classes. Start by asking your friends or health care practitioner for referrals or contact your local yoga teachers' association. Videotapes are okay for those with a good sense of body awareness, but I highly recommend you start with a good teacher in a class with no more than 15 students to insure some individual attention.

If you already attend a weekly yoga class, look for opportunities to practice daily without adding time constraints to your full schedule. Rising up on your toes slowly, and then gently back down makes the line at the grocery store go much more quickly, and it's far more peaceful than tapping your watch and worrying about running late. From how you walk, to the way you sit in your car, to how you perform your gardening tasks, if you do it with a straight spine you are practicing yoga.

27. Bicycling

I was rarely on a bike prior to my first trip to Europe in September, 2003. The Parisian women inspired me to get a one-speed girl's bike with upright handlebars, a wide seat and collapsible baskets on the back for groceries, wine and my yoga mat. Hey, if they can do their errands that way in a Chanel suit and heels, why can't I? Without the Chanel, of course.

It may not offer protection against osteoporosis since it's not load-bearing, but biking (known as cycling if you're serious about it) is a fun and simple way to increase your heart rate and get your blood pumping. One of the many benefits is being able to bike with your small children, spouse, friends or parents. Since the best sermon is a good example, it's a nice way to show those around you how to develop good exercise habits.

Biking is also beneficial to the Earth. If you bike to work just once a week you know you're helping to reduce the millions of tons of automotive pollutants going into our air and water. But my number one reason to use my bike for running errands and going to yoga classes is because it makes me smile.

With a bike, start simple. If you don't own one, look for a used one at a garage sale or in your local newspaper. Especially for the changing bodies and desires of children, used bikes are inexpensive and plentiful. When you're ready for an upgrade, check the bulletin boards at your local college a few weeks prior to the end of a term. Someone else's urgency or emergency can provide economic relief to your pocketbook. But don't scrimp on a helmet as it may save your life.

Biking shorts are okay if you're getting serious about this, but let's face it—they didn't earn the name "sausage pants" for nothing. My tree trunk legs need something more flattering, though I draw the line at the high heels I saw gracing the pedals of those women in Paris. I usually wear street clothes when biking since I use it for transportation.

When adjusting your seat, make sure it's low enough to provide a slight bend in your legs, but high enough to feel like a grown-up. I prefer the old-fashioned bikes that don't require you to lean way over in front; sitting upright is more comfortable and easier on the spine. The handlebar can make a big difference, too. If there's a little dip in the middle, effectively raising the handles, it brings you into a more upright position than with straight handlebars.

28. Dancing

Dear Freda, the London-born mother of one, was one of my very first clients. She was so passionate about dancing that after she was diagnosed with lung cancer, dancing again was her number one priority. Thankfully, we helped her achieve that goal prior to her passing in 2007. I miss her.

Dancing as a type of body movement feels more like fun than exercise. From the tango to the mambo to the twist to the unnamed dance you do in the privacy of your living room—all will provide some cardiovascular exercise and, even better, make you smile. For years I have done a little dancing while vacuuming or dusting to the tunes of the Rolling Stones, the Beatles or Beethoven. In addition to being a form of exercise, it's also very creative and can be a nice way to connect with your significant other if he or she is willing. Kids love dancing, too. They don't even know it's good for them and you may be able to get them to use a dust cloth at the same time. Sometimes I'll dance after returning from a walk with my husband when I want more exercise than he does.

Do you feel like you have two left feet? Check into classes offered at your local community college, recreation center or a dance studio. You may feel a little self-conscious when you first walk in, but guess what? So does everyone else. If you have more money than courage, arrange for private lessons.

If you live in Nebraska or Iowa, you may be lucky enough to be invited to a wedding reception complete with polkas, shots of whiskey and the interesting custom of pinning a $20 bill on the bride's gown, thereby ruining an expensive wedding dress. These "Dutch Hops" are a lot of fun—yes, I have first-hand experience—and if you dance enough you might negate some of the effects of the whiskey shots they continually pass around. In my experience, it's the German-Russian farmers who really know how to kick up their heels at a wedding reception.

Regardless of the technique, this is a pretty painless way to get your exercise. And here you thought this book was just for weekend warriors and health club honeys!

29. Swimming

For those recuperating from a long-term illness or who have concerns about too much jarring of the body, swimming is an excellent choice. It does not have the bone-building benefits of load-bearing exercise, but it can provide a terrific cardiovascular workout for your entire body. If stamina is a problem, or if you have limited use of your arms, start by using a kickboard. Although this method won't develop your upper body, it can be a perfect way to start—especially if you're recovering from a mastectomy or other surgery.

Like other forms of exercise, start slowly with just a lap or two. Even if you're fit from other activities, the occasional swim will likely leave you breathless in a short time. Take a short break in between laps or even half-way to help you recuperate during a longer workout. For those who know several different types of strokes, incorporating a variety can make the workout more enjoyable. The breaststroke takes the most energy, while the sidestroke can be a fairly relaxing way to get your breath back after you start to fade. Is the backstroke your favorite, but you're concerned about running into the edge of the pool? Ask whether a rope guide is available for installation over the pool to remind you when to stop.

If you never learned how to swim, don't despair. My grandmother took lessons at age 74 and quickly was able to do enough swimming to stay fit and enjoy herself. Perhaps this is why she lived to be 97!

Inquire about swim lessons through your local parks and recreation department or your regional chapter of the Red Cross. Often there are classes available for adults just like you. In addition to learning a new form of exercise, it may even save your life to know how to swim. And there's nothing more fun than splashing around the pool with your children, grandchildren, nieces, or nephews.

Equipment needs are minimal; a sturdy swim suit and towel is all that's necessary. You may prefer swimming with goggles, especially if you wear contacts. If you're concerned about the chlorine turning your hair a different color, invest a few dollars in a swim cap. Finding a pool to use can be as easy as contacting your local senior center or YMCA.

30. *Tips for Travelers*

Do your best to stick with your routine while away from home. You can usually walk on city streets, in airports, and through parks and shopping malls. Perhaps you can take a walk with a business associate instead of sitting in an office. If you like to work out in health clubs, make arrangements when you book your lodging. If there's not a gym within the hotel, guests often have access to one that is close.

Take a favorite workout tape with you or tune in to one of the many TV programs early in the morning. Too busy to take a formal exercise break? Make the effort to climb the stairs rather than using an elevator or walk to some of your appointments. One nice thing about big cities is that there is often a lot of walking involved just to reach your destination.

Airports are actually one of my favorite places to practice yoga and I love the funny looks I get while practicing a headstand. Yoga and/or stretching during or after your travel day is a great way to regain your equilibrium after the rigors of travel. If you bend forward to touch your toes (or shins), be sure to bend your knees and rest your ribcage right on top of your thighs. You'll be sure to get a good stretch without compromising your back. You can even stretch one arm at a time overhead while in your plane seat and do a little twisting there, or wiggle your bum occasionally on a long (or short) distance drive.

As always, drink lots of water. Three quarts a day is best while traveling; it's easier if you keep a water bottle with you at all times. And take some nuts and a couple of pieces of fruit to insure some good nutrition on travel days.

31. Preventing Joint Pain and Replacement

Betty, age 72, came to see me about joint pain that was keeping her from her two favorite activities: gardening and horseback riding. Within two weeks of modifying her diet and including both a teaspoon of cod liver oil and a daily quart of nettle tea (#58), she was virtually pain-free—even though she hadn't yet been able to give up her daily pack of cigarettes. This is a great demonstration of the power of using food as medicine.

An estimated 47.5 million adults suffered with chronic joint symptoms in 2001, and two million of these adults had to limit their daily activities due to pain. Despite this, 10.3 million adults with chronic joint symptoms have not visited a doctor for treatment. They may be the smart ones. The last thing you want is to consistently mask the problem with Band-Aid drugs because that is often all a doctor has to offer. Use those drugs judiciously for joint pain while continuing to address the underlying causes.

Arthritis is an inflamed joint, anywhere two bones meet in the body. When joints become arthritic, swelling causes stiffness, rigidity and tissue damage. It's a vicious cycle; as mobility decreases, the muscles surrounding the joint also weaken and deteriorate, allowing further joint damage. Eventually, your cartilage, ligaments and tendons suffer, too. The inner lining of the joint has a grease-like substance called the synovial fluid which reduces friction and allows freedom of movement. If the joint begins to malfunction, it's common to also experience a loss of synovial fluid which makes matters even worse.

While rare types of arthritis can be attributed to genetics, most who suffer can find improvement without drugs or surgery. Rheumatoid arthritis is actually an autoimmune disease, which means your immune system attacks itself; it is more complicated to heal than osteoarthritis, which is the type usually associated with aging. But rather than the aging process being the culprit, it's usually decades of poor dietary habits and lack of exercise. If you carry extra weight, that definitely exacerbates the problem.

Listen to your body's cry for help; start making some lifestyle changes to heal the cause of the problem. The human body is self-healing when given the right tools. Both rheumatoid arthritis and osteoarthritis respond beautifully to the suggestions below.

Nutrition and Joints

Do you remember the two biggest dietary contributors to inflammation from Chapter One on nutrition? Processed grains and sugar. Refined carbohydrates, and sometimes even whole grains, can aggravate and even cause degeneration.

Quality fats can reduce inflammation, so the low-fat diet hoax has made another contribution to disease. Excess omega-6 and omega-9 fats, most commonly found in commercially-raised beef, will add fuel to the fire of arthritis. However, consuming more fish will help dampen the flame. Yes, you can buy a fish oil supplement, but the real thing is better—and different from cod liver oil which I do recommend in small quantities for Vitamins A and D. Grass-fed beef is a much better choice than commercial as it has a natural balance of omega fats, and is usually free of hormones and antibiotics.

Because dehydration is also a major contributor to these symptoms, be sure to include two to three quarts of water daily—plus your nettle tea (#54). Walking around on dry joints is just as dreadful as it sounds.

Alignment, Balance and Exercise

When the tires on your car are misaligned, they wear unevenly. The musculoskeletal system operates the same way. The vast majority of people in our culture have muscular imbalances. This occurs when the muscles are tighter or stronger on one side of the body than they are on the other.

This dysfunction can occur by sitting at a computer, using one hand or arm predominantly, or letting one hip consistently drop while standing rather than being balanced on both feet. If you stand in front of a mirror, close your eyes and jump up and down a few times before opening your eyes; you will then see your true posture. Is one hip or shoulder higher than the other? Do you have "turtle head syndrome," in which your chin is jutted out over your chest? These points of imbalance get overused and contribute to damaging your joints and vertebrae.

For alignment issues, I suggest a good chiropractor and/or a therapeutic yoga instructor. Running and playing basketball are both hard on your joints, so walking and yoga may be your best forms of exercise as you age.

Susan's Simple Tip

Consider the "Paleolithic Posture" our forebears
had as they walked along the Earth with
unknown tree roots, etc. just under the surface.
They always had a slight bend in their knee,
rather than completely straightening the limb
as we now can easily do on concrete sidewalks.
Instead, keep that little bounce in your step to
protect both your knee and hip joints; it'll keep
you smiling, too.

Chapter Three

How Sex and Meditation Can Get You to the Same Place— And Other Lifestyle Tips

"Getting my lifelong weight struggle under control has come from a process of treating myself as well as I treat others in every way."

Oprah Winfrey
O, The Oprah Magazine, August 2004

Sandra was 31 when she came to see me about infertility after several years of following the advice of her physicians, unfortunately with frustrating results. She had been able to conceive once with the help of fertility drugs, but it was an ectopic pregnancy where the egg is fertilized in the fallopian tube rather than the uterus. The fallopian tube bursts in that situation, cutting any chances of future conception by 50 percent. Sandra's remaining fallopian tube also became blocked at times due to another health issue. Therefore, she tried IVF (in vitro fertilization) with two eggs being implanted, but that expensive procedure failed, too. Like many in her situation, she blamed herself for her inability to bring a child into this world and felt time was running out since her husband was 44 and running out of patience.

Even though there are herbs to "increase fertility," that's rarely where I start. Some women are so busy, they need to make space for a baby in their lives first—but that was not Sandra's issue. I felt confident that a combination of stress and a lack of minerals in her diet were limiting her already-compromised ability to conceive and carry a child to term. She had just started practicing yoga and reported it was helping her to relax; so I suggested she continue with yoga, drink a daily quart of strong red clover tea for critical nutrients, and set aside at least five to ten minutes a day for quiet time or meditation. I also suggested minor changes in her diet by adding some quality animal foods, more vegetables, and more quality fats. Thankfully, she conceived within four months and had a happy, healthy baby without complication.

Those little everyday choices we make with food, moving our bodies and managing our stress level can make a big difference.

32. Squeeze Your Creative Juices Every Day

While attending my first herbal medicine conference in 1997, I had the pleasure of hearing Terry Willard, Ph.D. speak on the value of creative expression to one's health. Terry, a highly respected Canadian herbalist, discovered that his clients were more likely to see improvements if they did something creative in their daily lives. I have found this to be true in my practice, as well.

Our ancestors had to be creative just to survive; their creativity involved necessities such as making tools, weaving cloth and forming baskets to carry food. They also had many festivals throughout the year, sometimes as many as 30 to 50 annually, which helped ease tensions from their daily effort to survive.

Consider the following creative expressions for a daily stress release:

◆ Singing or whistling, either with music in the background or all on your own.
◆ Doodling while on a telephone call with someone who has difficulty ending the conversation.
◆ Dancing while you dust. Play the Beatles or Bach, whatever makes your heart sing, and dance to the music while you're picking up the house or cleaning that glass door one more time.
◆ Journaling has been shown to be a powerful healer. If you tend to write down the negatives in your life, make it a point to write down five

things each day you're grateful for (#43 provides Gratitude Journal how-to's).
◆ Drawing or painting is an area where we're often self-critical, but for this purpose it doesn't matter if you do or don't have talent—just sketch something you find beautiful or interesting.

The release you will discover with these creative expressions will actually help you slow down, decrease stress and improve the results of your healthy choices.

Susan's Simple Tip
No time for creativity, you say? The vast majority of us spend time driving a car or using public transportation on most days. Sing to the radio while running errands or do some drawing or writing while in the bus, train or cab.

33. Meet Your Neighbors

Being a neighbor is a lost art in our hectic, garage-door-opener world. Since we don't even see each other as we're pulling into our respective nests, we rarely connect. The result is greater stress, isolation and complication in our lives. I've heard about a family who lost everything they owned when a stranger pulled up with a moving van, loaded their entire household and drove away without any questions being asked. Even if something this extreme never happens to you, there are still many benefits to having some type of relationship with your neighbors.

Just yesterday, our neighbors asked us for help while they're out of town. Picking up their car from the airport shuttle a few blocks away, watering plants a couple of times and taking their car back to the shuttle point on their return date is not a big deal. If this is something you don't have time for, please see Chapter Seven on Time Savers—you're too busy!

One of the benefits of doing these small tasks for our neighbors is their willingness to return the favor when we're out of town. Another neighbor of ours has two cats. Since we have a cat also, I'm happy to feed and stroke her cats twice a day when she's gone, and I know the favor will be returned. In all the years I've had a pet, I've never had to take one to a kennel. There is no one better suited to care for your pet than an 11-year-old neighbor—old enough to be responsible, but not old enough to instantly think about having a party while you're gone.

Besides trading favors while out of town, there are additional benefits from knowing your neighbors. For starters, you might actually like them and develop a satisfying friendship. Being friends with people who live close by is more conducive to entertaining spontaneously. If you and your neighbor are outside working in the yard, there's nothing more natural than getting together for a beer or glass of iced tea at the end of the day. Maybe you'll even learn how to have people over with a less-than-Martha-Stewart approach. If you live in an apartment or condo, consider a building-wide trick-or-treat for Halloween or some communal decorating for the holidays.

Do you pride yourself on being frugal and organized? Create a community co-op for the more expensive lawn-care tools. Snow blowers, lawn mowers, trimmers and hedge clippers are all used so infrequently, it would benefit everyone on your block to pool resources. Other possibilities include car pools, asking for help if you're under the weather, borrowing an egg or promoting a home-based business.

So what does all of this have to do with your health? Since at least 80 percent of all diseases have a stress component, anything you can do to "chill" will have a positive impact on your health. Knowing who to call for a babysitter or watchful eye while you're out of town will certainly help you feel more relaxed. If you're lucky, you might even make a friend or two.

Susan's Simple Tip

One ritual of the 1950's and 1960's I miss is the extension of kindness to a new neighbor. If time's too short to bake something, pick up a flavorful marinara sauce and some fresh pasta, with a small chunk of fresh, Romano cheese. Even a bunch of flowers from your garden or the florist can mean a lot to the new family on your block or in your apartment complex.

34. Quit Comparing Your Insides to Their Outsides

There are many aspects to health: mental, emotional, spiritual, and physical. If you want to improve both your mental and emotional health, stop comparing yourself to others. When you realize how often you do this—in so many ways—you'll be astounded. Ironically, you're not even making an accurate comparison since you're comparing your insides to others' outsides.

Let's take body physique as an example. When was the last time you compared the way your body looks to the way someone else's body looks? If you're a woman, I'll bet it was less than 24 hours ago. You know everything about your body—what it looks like naked, how it performs in terms of sports and everyday living, and whether it has problems with digestion, sleep, or cancer.

Not only have you carried this body around all your life, you've inspected it head to toe in a more scrutinizing manner than that of a lover. So you're aware of each and every flaw. Now what about that body you're comparing yours to; any idea whether it's healthy? Believe me, some of the thinnest people are terribly out of balance when it comes to health. Would you really trade your body for someone else's, not having any idea whether they might have cancer, AIDS or daily heartburn?

This inside/outside comparison stretches a lot farther than just your jean size. How about income, success of your spouse or kids, emotional problems, abilities in the kitchen or bedroom or general happiness and contentment in your life—ever compare yourself to another using *these* score-cards? Whenever you do, it's without knowing the full story. Maybe your acquaintance does drive a gorgeous car, wear beautiful clothes draped over an athletic body, have *seemingly* perfect kids, and a high-powered prestigious job with a six-figure income. What would you be willing to trade in order to have any of those things? Even if your life is in a deep valley right now, others have their own challenges which are rarely apparent. This same person may have a dreadful relationship with her parents, teenagers threatening to run away or experimenting with drugs, a husband who's cheating on her, and a life-threatening disease (probably from that high-stress, high-paying job). How appealing does her life sound now?

None of us knows for sure what goes on in someone else's life, and even if it really is good, you can't jump into their shoes. So how about trying to make your own more comfortable? If you've often fallen into the "comparison trap," use it as a wakeup call to make healthier choices, like eating more fruits and veggies or exercising regularly. Then once you've used that incentive, let go of comparisons as much as possible. Not only will you be healthier, but you'll save a lot of aggravation and money. Do you buy a new car every two years, or think you have to move into a larger home just to look like other, seemingly more "successful" people? It's expensive to "keep up with the Joneses"; they have their own problems, I assure you.

35. Create a Broad Support System

Once you get "real" about everyone having their own set of problems, you'll be in a better frame of mind to create a broad support system. The value of my support system was apparent to me as soon as it was threatened.

In April of 1996 I received my certification as a Master Herbalist and was simultaneously laid off from the Internet start-up company where I'd been working for two years. As their third employee, I was promised that if we made it big, I'd be richly rewarded. During my first year there as Director of Marketing, I loved it—even though I felt like a slacker for "only" working 60 hours a week. But the company never felt the same after the venture capitalists took control; so the layoff was perfect, right? Losing my job paved the way for me to establish my practice as an herbalist, while working part-time selling upper-end furnishings to pay the bills.

However, being laid off never feels good—even when many others are asked to leave—so I decided to rent my two favorite sad movies to help me work through it: *Beaches* and *Steel Magnolias*. Those classics helped me release the tears and feeling of rejection, so that a few days later, I could embrace my new career as an herbalist and health coach, as well as my new status as a recently divorced single parent.

The test came a few weeks later when a headhunter called with a job offer of over $100,000 from another Internet start-up—more money than I'd ever made, by far. The catch was the company was located in a community two hours away. It would require a move for me and my daughter to a new city where I knew no one. Turning the job down was initially easy since I was—and am—passionate about helping others heal. But a week later, financial fear kicked in and I found myself wondering if I had made a mistake. On further deliberation, I realized the price of leaving behind my support system was far too high, especially as a single parent. I needed to know there were friends I could call on in a crisis. And that start-up company could have gone belly-up in six months—along with the juicy salary.

Having others to lean on for support is critical because we all go through tough times and, even though we have to get through them ourselves, we don't have to do it alone. One of my biggest concerns with clients who are middle-aged and older is when they rely on their spouse/partner or just one friend for 100 percent of their social life and support.

This is not healthy at best and can be risky; whom will you turn to if that one person dies or leaves? As love and comfort deepen over time, it's easy to rely on that one person for all of our activities. Realistically, this can leave you feeling bereft and lonely at some point—and more susceptible to health problems. In the case of marriage, for example, most women outlive their husbands. If this could be you eventually, develop a broader support system using these ideas:

- ◆ Feeling rusty at socializing? There really is safety in numbers. Start by making a list of those people you have met who you might enjoy

knowing better. If that stumps you, start a page
in your day planner or journal where you can add
people to a list as you meet them. I started a
semi-annual tradition I call the "Wild and
Wicked Women's Gathering." The name isn't
important; what's important is that twice a year
we connect with each other. I include many
people I don't have time to see regularly but still
want in my life. We laugh, tell stories, share
parenting tips, and network in a gentle and
supportive way.

Susan's Simple Tip
This is not a Martha Stewart party. I ask each
person to bring a bottle of wine or snack to
share, but I also tell them to just bring themselves
if it's one of those tough days. Using wine glasses
I rent and return without washing and a simple
arrangement of flowers, the emphasis is on the
personal interaction—not the fu-fu.

◆ A gathering like the one described above will
provide you with many people with whom you
can make individual appointments for lunch, tea
or a walk in the park. Some will be flattered you
called and may be looking for the same type of
connection. Your one-on-one time doesn't have

to take up a lot of hours; a glass of wine after work or going for a walk, which you are hopefully doing anyway, are just a couple of options. Be creative.

◆ Serving on various non-profit boards has benefited me in many ways. It feels good to give back and is actually part of my health "prescription" to some people. If you're preoccupied with health issues, there is nothing like donating time to others less fortunate in order to remember all you have to be grateful for. And it's a way to meet like-minded people who may become friends or helpful business associates.

Some boards make it a priority to have a variety of occupations represented. This not only provides diverse points of view for healthy discussion, but also gives the institution a wealth of talent to draw from. The same principle holds true for us individually. When you need a good banker, CPA, physician, dentist, dry cleaner, plumber or attorney, it feels good to call someone reliable you know or who has been referred to you by a friend.

36. Smile

You may have heard it takes more muscles to frown than smile, but did you know it can actually reduce your stress level? Try it. Notice how you're holding your facial muscles right now; neutral at best, I'm guessing. Now smile, just a little. I know this feels foolish, but doesn't it immediately make you feel better? Often you'll notice yourself thinking of something positive as soon as you smile.

Deborah Benton has written books on the power of making a positive first impression. One of her recommendations is to always have the corners of your mouth "smile-ready" with the corners turned up just a bit. You look more open and receptive to new ideas; but more importantly, it helps you see life more positively. As a bonus, those little lines above your upper lip fade—at least temporarily.

For parents, smiling is even more important. Children hear "no" approximately 10-20 times more frequently than "yes." Is it any wonder two-year-olds get carried away with the word "no"? When parents smile more often, they tend to be more receptive to their children's ideas and look for ways to say "yes," which is great practice for saying "yes" to life. Some of the things we are most resistant to and fearful of, turn out to be life's greatest gifts. Be ready for them with a smile.

Turning the corners of your mouth up has significant health benefits, as well. Since it automatically puts you in a more positive frame of mind, smiling will help you see creative solutions to stressful problems. This, in turn, can actually lower your blood pressure and strengthen your immune system. Smiling also encourages you to stand straighter, opening your heart to new possibilities. Good posture is key to preventing or healing back and shoulder problems and will encourage you to walk with just a hint of an attitude. This is a great starting point for learning to be selfish.

37. *Choose to Be Selfish*

I admit it, I'm selfish—if the definition includes setting boundaries, saying "no" to the things I don't want to do, and saying "yes" to what makes me happy. It has taken me many years to learn "self care" which many people call "selfish." Previously, every non-profit organization in town knew just who to call when they were desperate. The result was me saying "yes," scrambling frantically to shove a new commitment into an already crowded schedule, and then feeling resentful when I had to say "no" to myself or my family.

Start searching for your motives behind saying "yes." If you say "yes" on a regular basis because you feel obligated, you will be saying "no" to the things that mean the most to you. Let's take a look at some examples and determine whether it's truly selfish to say "no" or if saying "no" would be a form of self care:

◆ The PTA at your child's school calls and asks you to spend time promoting a project you really don't believe in.

◆ Your church asks you to be in charge of the Christmas pageant this year—again.

◆ You made a commitment to help someone move, but the day before the moving date you come down with a wretched case of strep throat.

◆ Your husband asks you to pick up his dry cleaning which would be your ninth errand for the day and is very much out of your way.

◆ Your chosen political party needs a local chairperson at the last minute because the person who signed up has bailed.

Now I'm not suggesting you reject every plea for help; only that you consciously *choose* where you want to spend your time. Otherwise, these are the things that suffer:

◆ time with your kids, spouse or friends
◆ your new, and therefore fragile, exercise program or meditation practice
◆ the time it takes to feed yourself well with whole foods
◆ sleep
◆ sanity

Susan's Simple Tip

The past few years, my rule of thumb has been to only take on a new commitment when I consciously choose what to give up to allow time for it. The way I do that is by not saying "yes" immediately. I tell the caller I'll need to review my commitments to determine whether there is something I can give up to make the time necessary. Of course, this assumes you're not sitting around eating bon-bons while you watch the soaps. If you are, please contact me immediately as I thought that was a lost art.

The other thing that has helped me make better choices came from Oprah, our "Queen." She suggests only committing ourselves to those things we can truly feel excited about doing. If it doesn't excite you, pass. If you say "yes" due to duty and obligation, not only will you and your life suffer, but you will not do as good a job as someone whose heart sings when they contribute in this way. If we get enough hearts singing, more people will find creative solutions to problems rather than lashing out in violence.

Simple Tip
"No is a complete sentence."

Elisabeth Reinnersman,
My Spiritual Guide and Dear Friend

38. Do Everything 10 Percent Slower

Think of the last time you stubbed your toe, spilled the juice, locked your keys in your car, or bumped into a big stack of papers, spilling them to the floor. Chances are these incidents could all have been prevented by slowing down. We're all familiar with the concept, and many of us have tried to slow down, but with what degree of success? I tried and failed many times until I heard Judith Lasater, a fabulous yoga teacher, suggest we do everything just 10 percent slower. It has made all the difference for me as I attempt to create a saner world around me. Now when I find myself rushing, I say to myself "Just 10 percent; that's all I ask."

It felt overwhelming to "slow down," but 10 percent is finite and therefore, manageable. So the next time you feel frustrated or incur a small injury or create a terrible mess just at the most stressed and time-stretched moment, remember: "just 10 percent." You can do that!

39. Go Ahead and Drink—Wisely

Have you fallen into the "latest study" trap? I used to until I started asking, "Who paid for this study?" Even though I like to quote a few myself, a research project can be found to support almost any point of view, and the ones which reach the front page of your local newspaper are usually contradictory. First, you're told alcohol is bad for you; then, the next study "proves" red wine in moderation is good for you due to all those beta-carotenes (which incidentally, we can get from fruits and vegetables, too). Next, we hear that any alcohol raises our chances of getting breast cancer, shortly followed by the advice that moderate drinking (one or two beers or glasses of wine) each day can lower our chances of having a heart attack.

What's the best approach? Using some old-fashioned common sense will serve you well. Start listening more closely to your body every time you have a drink. If alcohol is bad for you, you'll feel a little sick or nauseous every time you have a drink. I used to feel like that every time I ate those little powdered sugar donuts, but I stopped when the light bulb came on about how they made me feel after eating them.

If your body doesn't feel crummy after having a drink, my advice is to relax and enjoy alcohol in moderation. By that I mean one or possibly two drinks a day, and not every single day. Your motive for drinking is important. Do you like the taste, enjoy being social, or feel it's a lovely complement to a delicious meal? That sounds healthy. But if alcohol (or food or sex or drugs) is the only way you can relax, pay attention to that red flag.

Think before you drink, and by all means, take a les-son from teenagers who are infinitely wiser about using designated drivers than my friends and I were in the 1970's. And if you're worried about those same teenagers smoking a little pot occasionally on the weekends, take a hard look at how much you drink. It may not be politi-cally (or legally) correct, but from a *health* perspective I worry less about occasional pot-smoking than I do about the growing number of adults who need two or more cocktails at the end of every day just to unwind. If this sounds familiar and a bit scary, please see #41 and #42 on Meditation in this chapter, and #26 on Yoga in Chapter Two for much healthier ways to reduce stress.

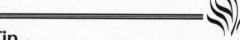

Susan's Simple Tip
For those of us working on keeping our weight in balance, it will help to ask your restaurant server to bring your wine or beer *with* the food, and bear in mind that alcohol is an appetite stimulant.

40. *Little Things That Make Life Easier*

When did you last feel frustrated and stressed because you couldn't find something—a pen, for example? Some details in life are inexpensively and easily handled when we let go of the way life "should" be. Especially when you live with children, it seems nothing stays in its designated spot for long. I was often in search of a pen or a pair of scissors until I realized how inexpensive they are and how easy it is to stock up. Pens are far less costly than therapy and massages, treatments that often feel like necessities when our lives are crazed.

Another simple tip to make life easier will be a big hit with your kids—free-for-alls. We established this weekly event years ago during a moment of panic at 6:00 P.M. when we opened the fridge with that age-old question: "What's for dinner?" Instead of allowing this end-of-the-day dilemma to increase your stress level, turn your family loose to fend for themselves. Leftovers are a natural, but your fussier family members may prefer scrambled or soft-boiled eggs, cheese and turkey on crackers, or a can of smoked oysters (my personal favorite). Sadly, few reach for a salad during a free-for-all, but if you're following the tip on getting more fruits and veggies into your diet (#2), one night a week won't deprive your body of nutrients. You can still sit together as a family or, if it's a completely crazed night, turn everyone loose to both cook *and* clean up after themselves (unless under the age of seven or eight).

A third way to ease your stress is to quit raking the leaves. Sounds radical, doesn't it? But in Europe, virtually no one sees this autumn activity as necessary. Perhaps it's motivated by our desire to keep up with the neighbors, but I actually found it rewarding to pull into our driveway recently and notice a very distinct line between our yard and that of our next-door neighbors. They clearly had worked diligently to rid their front lawn of every leaf, as was evidenced by an array of nature's compost material on our side of the green. Those leaves are just going to blow around again anyway, necessitating yet another Saturday morning of raking. So why not let them blow where they will, gently break down over the winter while protecting some of your plants, and then dig them out in the spring? Of course, this approach does depend on the quantity of deciduous trees in your yard.

When things are easily simplified—like stocking up on transparent tape, having a free-for-all dinner or letting the leaves blow—choose life's simpler path. The little things *do* make a difference. And all that money you save on therapy can go toward something more fun—like a vacation.

41. Mini-Meditations

With meditation, little tips can make a *big* difference. The word meditation often conjures up many false assumptions in the West. The truth is you don't have to be a Buddhist or Tibetan monk to derive significant health benefits from meditating. There are many studies now proving the link between regular meditation and lower blood pressure, lower cholesterol and fewer recurrences in heart attack victims. If you believe, as I do, that stress plays a role in at least 80 to 90 percent of all health problems, you'll be more open to meditation as a relaxation technique.

It helps to think of prayer as talking to God and meditation as listening. You've likely heard the old adage about the reason we have two ears and only one mouth. If you apply this concept to prayer and meditation, you'll see there may be a grand design at work. Instead of producing a heavy sigh at the thought of trying to find yet another 30 minutes in your day for something else you're "supposed to" do, get creative with your daily routine. Try some of these ideas for mini-meditations which won't take as much as an extra minute out of your day.

Driving

How much time do you spend in the car? Those who are lucky enough to avoid a nasty commute are still in the car most days. Why not use that time to create your own sense of peace rather than becoming stressed or angry with judgments about other drivers? Turn off the radio and count the number of breaths it takes for you to drive to the market, pick up the kids or make your way to the health club.

You'll be surprised how many times you need to start over with breath number one because you can't remember which number you're on! It's *good* to be distracted by any traffic issues needing your attention, but usually our distractions have more to do with our minds wandering. Gently bring the focus back to your breath and start over; think to yourself "inhale, one (as you exhale); inhale, two"; etc.

This simple technique helps train your mind to focus more and you'll quickly experience the benefits of deepening your breath. In addition to being more relaxed when you arrive at your destination, you'll find that practicing this regularly will actually lower your blood pressure and help you be a more relaxed, alert driver. Also notice your posture in the car. Are your knees in alignment with your hips and ankles? Do your bucket seats encourage your shoulders to round? Make adjustments for better posture while counting those breaths. A rolled up towel or small pillow behind your lower back can help counter the effect of bucket seats.

Stop Lights

How often do you drive through a yellow light just a little too late? Thousands of accidents are a result of this supposed time-saving technique. When my daughter was young, we struck a deal. Every third time I pushed a yellow light too far I had to buy her an ice cream. I also had to be honest about when I had done this without her in the car. Quite a few ice cream cones later, I got a lot better at preparing to stop when signaled to do so by the yellow light.

Now when I'm sitting at a red light, I use it as a reminder to focus on my breath or make conscious contact with my "Higher Power." It's even more effective when you turn off the radio.

The Market

What do you do while standing in line at the grocery store? Tap your foot, look at your watch, worry about whether your kids are killing each other at home or fret about being late for your next appointment? That's what most of us do, and if you're working on dying early from a heart attack, keep it up. But regardless of how you choose to use that time, you are in line and it certainly won't move any faster because you're late or worried or stressed.

As long as you're there, try closing your eyes for just a second or two in order to draw your attention inward. Then notice your breath. Are you breathing through your nose or your mouth? Is your breathing shallow or deep and full? Work on extending both the inhale and exhale a little longer. For further relaxation, make the exhale a little longer than the inhale. And LET GO.

If you want to practice yoga simultaneously, gently rise up onto your toes for a moment (unless you're wearing painful shoes). This will strengthen your legs, improve your balance and help you relax rather than feel stressed

while you're in line. Use this time productively for relaxation and you'll soon shift from stressed-out to smiling.

Downloads

Ever use a computer? They can be a major source of stress.
Massage therapists see more people with carpal tunnel
syndrome and shoulder and neck problems than ever
before. Even with a high-speed connection to the Internet, it's common to wait for several minutes while down-
loading a file or a "cookie."

What can you do besides tapping your foot? You
guessed it, focus on your breath. Count them or expand
them. Or while you're concentrating on your breath,
reach your arms and hands up toward the sky and then
try to drop your shoulders back down.

Cooking

Preparing nourishing food for those we love—that needs
to include you as well—is one of life's greatest blessings.
Especially if you don't expect the people you cook for
to be grateful. It's not just the olive oil and garlic that
make the Mediterranean diet one of the healthiest in
the world. Those who live in Italy, Greece and France
are more likely to see cooking as an act of love. Preparing, serving and savoring healthy food is an art in those
countries.

Through focusing on the love and care that goes into
your meals, you can actually make it a meditation. Sometimes I'll stand on one foot while resting the other on the
inside of my other calf (called Tree Pose in yoga), which
helps me stand comfortably for longer periods.

A lot of the meditation benefit from cooking can come from actually sitting down with the family to enjoy a meal together. And I'm intrigued with a study showing that the only common denominator among a group of honor-roll students was that they all sat down to eat with their family most nights at home. Have your child do a class survey and you'll learn how infrequently this occurs.

Waiting at Your Doctor's Office

When was the last time you didn't have to wait for your physician or dentist? You might commonly pick up the latest issue of *People* magazine to thumb through. This may be one of the ways you compare yourself to all those thin, beautiful, wealthy people whose photos are air-brushed and computer-doctored. Do you really need one more way to come up short?

Instead, go "inside" by closing your eyes (making the receptionist wonder a little) and as you inhale, try to create more space between your vertebrae, lifting the back of the head a little and keeping your chin parallel to the floor. Then when you exhale, drop your shoulders. Yoga practice has shown me how much tension many of us carry here. This movement will also reduce any "white-coat stress" you might experience when the nurse takes your blood pressure.

42. Deeper Meditation

If you'd like to be more deliberate and move into deeper meditation, start setting aside five to ten minutes first thing in the morning. Even if you have to get up earlier than usual, the payoff will be substantial. Start by reading a page out of your favorite spiritual book or one-page-a-day book, such as *Meditations for Women Who Do Too Much* by Anne Wilson-Schaef. This will help you center yourself and may be all you accomplish at first if you allow just five minutes.

So be it; starting is the hard part. Don't criticize yourself for only starting with five minutes a day. If you allow yourself an additional five minutes, sit comfortably with your eyes closed and feet on the floor. Notice the cycle of your inhales and exhales without forcing your breath in any way.

Next, start counting your breath backwards from number twenty-seven down to zero. Think to yourself, "inhale (as you inhale), twenty-seven (as you exhale); inhale, twenty-six" ...and so on down to zero. A teacher of mine from India said to start with the number twenty-seven because it is an auspicious number.

If you're like most of us, you'll notice your mind wandering. This is *normal.* If you beat up on yourself every time your mind wanders, you're defeating the purpose of meditation. When I trained for a week at The Chopra Center in California, I learned there are three things that can happen during meditation: falling asleep (indicating your need for more rest), having uninvited thoughts pop into your mind, and slipping into the "gap." The gap is the goal of meditation, but the other two things happen regularly for many people, especially uninvited thoughts. If falling asleep regularly is a problem, determine whether you're sleep-deprived, and seek help if you're unable to get enough rest.

After counting backwards from twenty-seven to zero, continue to relax in your sitting position as you keep your focus on your breath. As each thought intrudes, gently let it go and refocus on your breath. Jack Kornfield, author of *A Path With Heart*, suggests thinking about training your mind as you would a puppy. When paper training a new puppy, you'll have the most success if you gently bring him back to the newspaper each time he piddles somewhere else.

What response do you think you'd have if you beat that adorable puppy each time he urinated in the wrong place? Your mind also responds more effectively with gentle attention on your breath, rather than beating up on yourself for meditating "incorrectly" when thoughts arise. The Bibliography will guide you toward some good books if you want to explore meditation further. It is a wonderful practice full of health benefits—physical, mental, and spiritual.

Susan's Simple Tip

Do you struggle releasing all those thoughts and focusing only on your breath? Thich Nhat Hanh, acclaimed author and Buddhist teacher, suggests a mantra that I use often: "I have arrived, I am home." Say that to yourself with each full breath (one inhale, one exhale) as a reminder that "being" is enough.

43. Rely on God (Good Orderly Direction)

As a former Episcopalian, I hesitate to write this down, but discovering the "Middle Path" with spirituality has made such a huge difference in my life, I simply must share it with you. At the age of 14, I challenged my parents about the Bible being truly representative since it was only written by men, and left the church a few years later because I experienced more dogma and less of an actual relationship with a Higher Power (aka God). A true child of the 1960s; feminism hit me early.

My mistake was in throwing spirituality out with religion. It took years to uncover the possibility that I could have a personal relationship with God, using daily prayer and meditation. It not only made me a *better* person—it also made me a *happier* person. This does not mean I considered religion to be bad; it just wasn't a fit for me. If it works for you, that's great; but for those who feel uncomfortable with religion, it's important to explore personal choices that *do* work.

For me, this came about through the Al-Anon program which supports friends and families of alcoholics. At my first meeting, I was told that the program was about how I could take responsibility for my own life—not how to fix others around me. I didn't go back for six months. How could it have been *me* making my life miserable? What I learned after I went back is that my stress is usually about me and how I respond to things in my life, not about someone else who doesn't live up to my expectations. This was a hard pill to swallow for the "Queen of

Control," but I soon learned that the path to my peace is reflected in The Serenity Prayer:

> "God, grant me the serenity to accept
> the things I cannot change,
> The courage to change the things I can,
> And the wisdom to know the difference."

I'm not suggesting you rush out to join Al-Anon, though it can be helpful for many people. What I am proposing is that even if religion feels like putting your square peg into a round hole, spiritual healing is still available and from many sources. I can't guarantee that God or a Higher Power exists; all I can say is that when I believe it's true and act accordingly, my life goes better. Most of the time, the "Queen of Control" has abdicated her throne—and feels much happier and more peaceful as a result. I'm actually grateful now for the alcoholic in my life that prompted my association with Al-Anon since it helped me create a deeper spiritual connection.

44. The Gratitude Journal

For the few of you who don't watch Oprah, the gratitude journal is one of the greatest tips for peace of mind I can recommend. The queen of talk shows started talking about it a few years ago, so by now you may need a reminder to practice this even if you have heard about it. This is the way it works:

Every night before you go to sleep, write down five things you're grateful for. They don't have to be big things, but can be anything from the sun shining that day to your daughter telling you she loves you. Even when you're down in the dumps you can find five things that bring gratitude to your heart.

You will discover that there are many things to be grateful for, and your worries will start to lessen with that perspective. It's true that whatever we focus on expands; if you focus on all the small things that went wrong that day, you're likely to see more of them. But when you start to express gratitude for all the things in your life that are going well, you'll start to see your life in a more positive way, and create more positive outcomes.

A fancy journal isn't needed; before you put it off one more day, just use some scrap paper until you can pick up a little spiral notebook or journal. I write in mine off and on, and I've discovered a pattern with this process. When life feels good, I forget to write in the journal; but when new challenges come up, I start using it again and things start to turn around. It may be only in your own mind, but if you can create a more positive attitude for yourself, there is no limit to what you can do. Writing in a gratitude journal takes a couple of minutes each day, and offers a tremendous pay-off.

Susan's Simple Tip
Don't feel guilty if you only use this when life is tough and you're grasping at anything that might help. It's natural to ignore this tool when life feels blissful. Enjoy the bliss.

45. The Worry Journal

For those of you with a black belt in worrying, this tool could add years to your life. Studies show that fretting about those things beyond your control contributes to stomach ulcers, high blood pressure and heart disease. The heart is much more than a strong muscle beating thousands of times each day, pumping blood through your body. It is also the center of your emotions; hence the heart's vulnerability to worry, unresolved anger and resentment.

The worry journal concept was shared by a valued client who used this idea to successfully treat her chronic sinus infections. Strange as it may seem, your unresolved emotions lodge in your body's most vulnerable places. For some it will be the sinus cavities, for others the gastrointestinal system and still others will experience heart problems as a direct result of stress. The worry journal helps you let go of the things you worry about which are beyond your control—at least 95 percent of all you fret about. Here's the process:

- In a notebook or journal, draw two lines down your paper vertically to create three columns.
- Title the first column, "What I'm Worried About."
- Title the second column, "My Desired Outcome."
- Title the third column, "What I Can Do About It."

Make a list of all the different things you're worried about in the first column, and then write down the best possible outcome in the second column. If the third column produces the word "nothing" over and over, I suggest a modification. Provided you're willing to accept there is *something* out there wiser than you are, change the word "nothing" to "pray" and let go. There's a wonderful phrase used in Al-Anon (for families and friends of alcoholics): "If you pray, why worry? If you worry, why pray?" This is a great reminder that you are not the queen or king of the worry universe and you might as well toss out that crown and use your scepter as a walking stick.

If you need to go one step further than the worry journal, write down whatever is bothering you the most on a scrap of paper and place it in a "God Box." This can be a special container of your choosing; or if you can't make it to your God Box soon enough, just slip it into a handy drawer in your kitchen or desk. This is a physical way of "turning it over" to a power greater than yourself and is often accompanied by a big sigh of relief. If you're struggling with the word God, think of it as "good orderly direction."

I like the phrase "Higher Power" since most of us can relate to something greater than we are whether it's Mother Nature, the Universe or even the highest aspect of our collective selves. However you define it, tap into it and use it. Worrying is a destructive emotion—and gives you wrinkles before your time.

46. The Easiest and Most Effective Relationship Tools

Clearly, I will not be able to address your deepest, darkest relationship problems; that would take more than a 500-word tip. However, many problems with our loved ones can easily be mitigated before we start worrying and stressing about them. If you're contemplating divorce or any other drastic life-changing measures, it may be time to seek the care of a professional. If things aren't quite that dire, consider the following suggestions—these are some of the simplest, most effective problem-solving tools I've discovered:

- ◆ *Practice "Letting Go" as often as possible.* I love the phrase, "Everything I've let go of has claw marks down its back!" For those with control issues, letting go is a tall order—and an essential one for your health. The more we try to control people and things around us, the likelier we are to have stress-related illnesses. Using the God Box mentioned in #45 can be a helpful tool. Biting your tongue helps, too, but it hurts.
- ◆ *Give Support in "Their Currency."* It's common for us to give what *we* would like to receive rather than what the other person would experience as supportive. Men are actually pretty easy to figure out; they like to know that they're doing okay whether it's financial support, sex or a good golf swing. Women can often be easy to

figure out, too. Tell them they're beautiful, a great mom/wife/employee and express verbal appreciation for the eight million little things they do on a regular basis. But the only way to know for sure what your spouse/friend/coworker wants for support is to *ask* them. Then make a note in your day planner to offer that form of support a few days down the road so it will feel genuine to your partner. You'll be amazed at the results.

◆ *Practice the Three A's: Awareness, Acceptance and Action.* "Foot in Mouth" disease is common and it's difficult to take back something you've said, especially if it sounded cruel. Most of us, when we see or hear something that bothers us, immediately respond with an attack or criticism, sometimes cleverly disguised as helping the other person. Before immediately jumping from "Awareness" to "Action," try practicing "Acceptance" first—in silence. I prefer giving it 24 hours if possible before commenting on the transgression. This gives me time to determine whether it's truly important and how I can respond in a compassionate way. Usually I just forget about it or think to myself, "If this is the worst thing I can say about my husband, I'm lucky."

◆ *Say "Thank You" every day.* In a former marriage I was ridiculed at times for saying "thank you" a lot. The family I grew up in considered it normal to express thanks for little, everyday things.

When I was initially criticized for this, I
mistakenly concluded it was a defect of mine.
After further consideration, I concluded that
this is a wonderful trait. If more of us expressed
thanks to someone for unloading the dishwasher,
stopping to get the dry cleaning, fixing the
sprinkler head, or picking up the kids, I'm
convinced we would see a decline in divorce
statistics. The people we live with, and often
love the most, are the ones least likely to
hear "thank you." They are also the ones
most likely to benefit from it. The kicker is…
you will, too.

◆ *Ask for what you need.* "If he really loved me;
he'd *know* what I want!" Does this sound
familiar? I'm sad to say that women are especially
guilty of this one. Is your partner a psychic?
Probably not, and furthermore, he may be so
preoccupied with his work performance or last
bowling score that it hasn't even crossed his
mind you might be in need of a hug, a question
about how your day was, or whether little
Johnny's sore throat turned out to be strep.

For those who feel verbally challenged by
this task, consider using a deck of cards called
"Your Heart's Desire." The cards come with
two little easels (one for each side of the bed)
and say things like "I need a back rub" or "an
evening alone" or "my favorite position." It's
a fun and easy way to ask for what you need

from your partner. For ordering information call Sue Sell at 970-266-9147.

◆ *Practice "Forgiveness" in a new way.* My favorite definition of forgiveness is letting go of all hope for a different past. Think about it. When you are unable to forgive, it's usually *you* that is the loser. And that stockpile of resentment could contribute to cancer or something equally nasty. Many of us think of forgiveness in terms of making it okay for the other person to be a screw-up. When you practice forgiveness with a holier-than-thou attitude, you know you're in trouble. Instead, try to give up all hope for the past to be different 'cause (guess what?) all your anger will not change the past. Letting go is far more beneficial to *you* than it is to the one being forgiven.

47. The Joy of Sex

For those of you who looked through the Table of Contents and came here first...welcome! I hope that tapping into the energy of your sexual drive will lead you to other health tips in the book, especially #46 on relationship tools. Dr. Ruth I'm not, but from a Chinese medicine perspective, regular sexual activity can improve your health. In fact, herbalists in China suggest having sex two to four times a week for optimal health. The one caveat is that you need to enjoy it.

You'll find specific suggestions in Chapter Five, "Special Issues for Women," but why not start early with such a hot topic? Sex isn't everything, but it can often be a barometer of how well your special partnership, and your body, is working. If you have a good sex life, it probably accounts for five to ten percent of the importance of your relationship. If you *don't* have a good sex life that percentage feels like 90 percent.

For those who have been together many years and need a shift, I recommend a book called *How to Make Love to the Same Person for the Rest of Your Life...and Still Love It!* by Dagmar O'Connor. Part of what you'll find in this quick read is a set of instructions for bringing some spark back into your partnership that was—hopefully—present in your early days of dating.

Occasionally I'll ask my husband to pretend we're still dating which means more kissing, more foreplay and less urgency about achieving orgasm. That alone can work wonders. Or perhaps you need to start the foreplay with dinner out or a movie *without the kids*. Short on cash? Consider using or creating a baby-sitter co-op with your friends and neighbors to allow you and your spouse to attend a free concert in the park with a picnic basket. Time alone with your spouse is critical when your children are young, yet it is most often neglected by busy parents of small children.

Are you single and feeling left out of this discussion? Sex with yourself can easily move from masturbation to making love to yourself with the right shift in heart space. When I was single (again), I decided to stay uninvolved for a year—after strong encouragement from my therapist. This was especially good for me since I had been in relationship with a boyfriend or husband ever since the age of 14. But being in my 30's with that healthy sex drive thirty-something women are famous for, I soon learned to make good use of a woman's best friend—a vibrator.

A dear friend of mine had given me my first one for Christmas the previous year, and I'm amazed it took me so long to utilize this wonderful tool. It can also be helpful for menopausal women (and their husbands) who are finding it more difficult to achieve orgasm. One of my more conservative menopausal clients thanked me for suggesting a vibrator when orgasms became more difficult to achieve; she joked with me that the $90 she spent may have saved her husband from carpal tunnel syndrome!

There are no rules when it comes to sex as long as both partners agree, so don't hesitate to suggest new options. Especially for those who have been together a long time, mixing things up a bit might be just the ticket for a stagnant sexual relationship. However, if you are not

in a committed relationship (i.e. sexually exclusive) proceed with caution. A nurse once told me that my best
protection against sexually transmitted infections was
knowledge; knowing my partner and knowing he wasn't
having sex with anyone else. If you're single, consider
using the following as a guideline: only have sex with
someone who at least has the *potential* to be a long-term
or lifetime partner. The ten-date rule (before having sex)
can be helpful, too—even if you end up breaking your
own rule on date eight or nine. Be careful out there; the
life you save may be your own.

Susan's Simple Tip
There's nothing simple about understanding the
opposite sex.

48. Sleep

If you find yourself falling asleep while your partner is try-ing to arouse you, your body is telling you something: "More rest, please!" Most Americans are sleep-deprived. We can easily blame it on too much work or the growing needs of others (spouse/partner, kids, pets or friends). But rather than blame someone, which is destructive to all, focus on solutions and find the gifts present in your sleep problems.

For example, lack of sleep may be the nudge you need to set better boundaries with others. When you can't say "no", it's either sleep or family time that suffers. If your boss continually dumps more work on you than you can handle, just smile and say, "I'm happy to work on this project as soon as you let me know which of the other 14 projects you've given me in the past month can wait." Yes, it's best to be tactful…so ask your boss for guidance on which of your assignments has the highest priority. Or if you'd prefer not to have a boss at all, check out *The Four Hour Work Week* by Timothy Ferris.

All of us need to know how to set limits with those around us, but others rarely like it when we do—too bad! If we don't set boundaries we give our essence away; con-sequently we have nothing left over for those we love. See #37 if setting limits is a particularly challenging issue for you.

Doing what appears to be selfish is actually smart self care. Without it, finding enough time for sleep and rest doesn't happen. If you're still not getting a good night's sleep after setting boundaries and carving out enough time for the rest you need, try the following:

◆ Avoid watching news programs just before bedtime. Television is stimulating in general, but the news is particularly problematic due to the negative content. If it's a critical ritual for you, try watching an earlier news program or recording your late-night news to watch the next morning. The hour before bed needs to be spent in restful activities.

◆ Create a ritual of a nightly bath, complete with lavender essential oil (two to four drops) and a handful of Dead Sea bath salts which are often available in bulk at your health food store. A warm bath will soothe tension, relax your muscles and pave the way for a good night's sleep—and it's considerably cheaper than therapy. Add some candles and gentle music for a truly decadent get-away right in your own bathroom. Aaaahhhhhhhhhh.

◆ Reading just before bedtime is a good habit to get into, as long as the reading material is relaxing. Books on gardening, spiritual issues or creative endeavors will invite a good night's rest much more readily than a murder mystery. A good novel can fill the bill as long as it isn't so engrossing you can't put it down when it's time to turn out the light.

◆ Reduce your caffeine intake (a good idea anyway), especially after noon. Replace your afternoon coffee with green tea (Celestial Seasonings Green Tea with Berry Plum has proven acceptable to even the fussiest tea drinker) or a strong chamomile tea in the evening to help your body relax. Drinking enough water throughout the day can be helpful, too. Two quarts a day is necessary unless you're ill—then increase it to three to four quarts a day, depending on your size.

◆ Nettle tea counts toward your total water consumption and is usually the herb I suggest as a starting point for insomnia issues. Since it does so much to support often-depleted adrenal glands, it can be the perfect solution for those who wake up between 2:00 and 4:00 A.M. and are unable to go back to sleep. Waking at that time can also indicate a congested liver for which I often suggest milk thistle tincture and being in bed by 10:00 P.M.

◆ Other herbs can be helpful for sleep, but if you're on sleep medication, first seek guidance from your health care practitioner. Hops, passionflower, skullcap, blue vervain, California poppy and oat are all helpful. Valerian root is more commonly known for sleep inducement, but if you take more than the recommended dose it may actually keep you awake. I've also found it to be contraindicated for those with a ruddy complexion who tend to "run hot."

If you've tried almost all of these solutions without success, it's time for a physical evaluation by your health care practitioner before sleep deprivation further deteriorates your health. If you need to find a practitioner, see #49. Chronic insomnia is damaging; five months of only two to three hours of sleep a night gave me migraines and a few other entertaining symptoms. And yes, I was a nut case.

Thank goodness for nettle tea and Susun Weed who introduced me to it as a powerful, yet gentle, medicine.

Simple Tip

If you wake up during the night and have trouble going back to sleep, try making a mental "Gratitude List" and see how much faster you get back to sleep than when you obsess about all the items on tomorrow's to-do list. I also find that one-half to one teaspoon of an herbal formula works wonders: two parts passionflower, one part blue vervain and one part motherwort. After many years of trying various herbs for sleep issues, this combination has been most consistently effective for baby boomer, mid-life women who have sleep problems. Eureka!

49. Create Your Own Health Team

Even if you're 100 percent healthy now, it's smart to gather information prior to needing a health care practitioner in the future. Consider creating your own team: a skilled and open-minded physician, a massage therapist, an herbalist, a psychotherapist and a chiropractor. The best way to find qualified practitioners is through referrals from friends or from other practitioners you trust. If you have an acute need and don't know who to ask for a referral, start with the Yellow Pages but be armed with the following questions:

- ◆ What is your educational background?
- ◆ How long have you been practicing full-time?
- ◆ What is your general philosophy on health and healing?
- ◆ How much do you charge?
- ◆ Do you have any pro bono clients or a sliding scale for those who are financially challenged?

Take notes and pay attention to what your intuition is telling you, not only based on the answers but also on the person's voice and general demeanor. Since it's virtually impossible to get a physician on the phone, another alternative is to gather this information from their assistant or nurse—preferably someone who works directly with the doctor.

You want to ask how long they've been devoting their energies full-time to this work in order for you to learn about their experience and dedication, but be aware that it's sometimes necessary for new practitioners to work part-time for a year or two elsewhere while establishing their practice. I have first-hand experience with the challenges of starting an integrative medicine practice while providing for my daughter as a single parent.

Formal education is a mixed bag with practitioners of integrative medicine. Having some type of education as a foundation of knowledge is important, but I've known incredibly knowledgeable and helpful herbalists who have never been to herbal medicine school or pursued higher education. Instead, they sometimes train as an apprentice with an herbalist for years and study on their own. Herbalists in Europe, especially England, are usually much better educated from an academic and clinical standpoint since European countries view medical herbalism and modern medicine as equally valuable. Your best bet is finding a practitioner by referral from clients who have had positive experiences.

What you're looking for in a practitioner's healing philosophy is a holistic approach, which should include nutrition, exercise and lifestyle choices. If a practitioner sees healing through just a single focus on drugs, herbs, chiropractic adjustments, massage, or supplements, it's not inclusive enough for long-term healing. In my practice, I always search for the simplest and least expensive methods for healing first, then offer further suggestions or referrals as needed.

The pro bono question helps uncover their motivation for being a practitioner; hopefully it's to help others heal rather than just for the almighty dollar. Giving their services away for nothing (pro bono) is not a requirement, but they should at least offer adjusted fees for seniors and students, and many practitioners will consider trades. The common perception is that anything given away is not valuable; however, I look for a potential trade rather than charge nothing. This in itself has been healing to my clients who have a self-esteem crisis and can't think of anything they have to offer. While we explore their skills together we're getting them on the road to a healthier self-esteem.

When you start working with someone new, have a clear idea of what would make this association a success; then ask the practitioner if your expectations are reasonable. If someone isn't willing to spend five minutes with you on the phone to answer your questions, consider it a gift. Don't waste any further time with that person.

Once you start working with a new practitioner, be sure to give their suggested protocol a chance; implement their suggestions for at least three to four months before moving on. My one caveat on this is that if you don't feel comfortable for any reason when you first meet the practitioner, search for someone else. A sense of connection and trust with your primary care giver is vital for improving your health.

Bottom Line? Ask for referrals, trust your instincts and keep searching until you find the best fit. This is great life-training for asking for what you need.

Susan's Simple Tip
Keep a folder or file for all your medical tests and a list of supplements, herbs and pharmaceutical drugs you're currently taking. Not only will this be helpful to your health care practitioners, but it may be highly valuable if you have to make an urgent trip to the emergency room.

Chapter Four

My Favorite Herbs
for Healing and Prevention

"The doctor of the future will give no medicine, but will interest his patients in the care of the human frame, in diet, and in the cause and prevention of disease."

Thomas Edison, Inventor

Pam, a 49-year-old single mother of two teenagers called me in a panic. Her gynecologist had just informed her that the *only* solution for her excessive uterine bleeding—bleeding which had been flowing for three weeks straight—was a hysterectomy. Pam could not afford the surgery and had no health insurance. In addition, she was concerned about the many post-operative side effects and the time away from her fledgling business. Although I was unable to convince her to modify her diet and start a gentle exercise program, my herbal "friends" worked beautifully. Within two hours of starting her on an herbal tincture of yarrow and shepard's purse, Pam's bleeding started to lessen, and then completely stopped after 24 hours. And you thought herbs were always slow to work compared to drugs and surgery!

Plants are still relied on by 80 percent of the world's population as the first choice for healing—90 percent if you leave out the United States. Granted, many of that majority has little financial choice; but the truth is, plant medicine works. Laboratory research on herbs is on the rise, yet it's still true there is limited "scientific" evidence of plants' efficacy. Any guesses about why? There's very little profit to be made because Mother Nature's gifts cannot be patented by a drug company. Thank God.

Though scientific research on the effectiveness of herbal remedies is somewhat limited, we have hundreds to thousands of years of empirical evidence, "empirical" meaning "based on observation." In other words, we know what has worked for those experiencing particular health problems over the past centuries. This empirical evidence is every bit as valid as laboratory evidence. In my opinion, it's actually *more* reliable since the results are based on the use of the whole plant and its use with humans, rather than isolating the constituents *currently believed* to impact a health problem and studying only those constituents on rats in a laboratory. Both empirical evidence and laboratory evidence, however, are helpful and both need to be valued and used.

Compared to herbal medicine, modern medicine is the new kid on the block, coming on the scene as it did about 1900. It provides helpful diagnostic tools plus the ability to respond quickly and well to emergency first-aid needs. But just because we have certain new tools at our disposal, such as complex pharmaceutical drugs with a host of potential negative side effects, doesn't mean we should always use them. Isolating one physical imbalance, without being aware of the body and person as a whole, rarely fosters true healing. To make things worse, not only has medicine become too complicated, the associated costs are out of reach for most of the world's population— even for those *with* health insurance.

Please don't blame the physicians for this reduction- ist view of health. Many became doctors for all the right reasons but were molded by workaholic-mentality med- ical schools that also came with huge price tags. Many doctors I know are overworked and less well-paid than a decade ago. This is often due to HMOs and insurance companies dictating how, when and with which tools physicians can treat their patients. We, the consumers, got into the habit of demanding a quick fix and handing over the responsibility for our bodies and our health to the health care system—right along with a check. We had faith that these physicians, anointed by God, could take care of us. As we take back our bodies, it's up to us to decide what to put into them, and to know the potential side effects of those choices.

Though many in the West are skeptical about the efficacy of herbs because of limited scientific validation, more and more are experimenting with them because of their frustration with the ineffectiveness and negative side effects of pharmaceuticals. Part of the skepticism about herbal medicine is a result of consumers choosing herbs from an overwhelming array of choices at their local health food or drug store. Receiving advice from an $8 an hour employee, who may have little or no training and spends only two or three minutes with you, often leads to unimpressive results. Add to that the probability that you're buying a pill or capsule that may have lost much of its potency after sitting on the shelf too long, and you can see why success may be limited.

Working with a trained herbalist is your best assurance of success with herbs. If that's not possible for you, this chapter will provide guidelines for safe self-medicating. I have included the plants I reach for most often in my dispensary, plus those which have many uses for common, everyday ailments. There are many Materia Medicas available that list a hundred or more herbs in detail. I've included some in the Bibliography.

The herbs listed in this chapter are inexpensive, easy to obtain, and easy to use with only a few notes of caution. In a perfect world, you would prepare them yourself, either in tincture form (an alcohol extract) or a tea. But given the Blackberry-driven lives of many, I will also tell you how to buy them ready-made.

Using a little common sense, you can experiment with these herbal remedies for yourself and your family with virtually no negative side effects. However, with more complicated health issues, or if you use any prescription pharmaceutical drugs, please follow my suggestions in #49 to find a qualified herbalist, or a naturopathic physician who is well-educated in the use of herbs.

50. Which Is Better—Drugs or Herbs?

Why do Americans think that modern medicine and herbal medicine are "alternatives"? Be wise; use the best of both worlds. Modern medicine for diagnostics and emergency first aid; food, exercise and herbs for prevention, vitality and improving most health problems; modern medicine again when you just have to have a Big Gun. An example of a necessary Big Gun is insulin for those with Type I diabetes.

As mentioned previously, I value the diagnostic tools and first-aid abilities of modern medicine, but I am not a proponent of most pharmaceutical drugs. Because that industry is consistently fueled by the almighty dollar, I'm skeptical of virtually any drug created in a laboratory. I am not anti-physician, but I am very anti-pharmaceutical. If you start to ask for the PDR (Physicians' Desk Reference) listing for any drug prescribed by your doctor, you will be astounded at the number of potential side effects. Even though the FDA (Food and Drug Administration) requires expensive testing before granting approval for a new drug, consumers are still the guinea pigs.

There is also an unhealthy relationship between the pharmaceutical companies and physicians. In addition to limited physician education regarding side effects, some of the HMO's actually *pay the doctors more for prescribing certain drugs.* Sounds a lot like a kickback to me.

Recall the last time you read a story in your local newspaper about a new drug approved by the FDA. Most articles inform you of the many possible benefits of that drug with little mention of potential side effects. How long after it's on the market might you read about concerns regarding the negative side effects of that same drug? Often, not until a number of deaths or major health problems have occurred—directly related to that pharmaceutical— has the drug company been forced to remove it from the market. This is a common scenario, and an unacceptable "side effect."

It is important to be aware of potential herb-drug interactions, and I always take this into consideration with new clients. Negative interactions with legal drugs are the most common origin of reported problems with herbs. But when did you last read about drug-drug inter-actions? Many Americans, especially seniors, are on three, five, even ten different medications. And several were likely prescribed to "alleviate" side effects from one or more of the previously prescribed drugs.

Since herbs are mistakenly labeled as the new kids on the block—even though they've been used for thousands of years—the media quickly exaggerates potential prob-lems, while often remaining silent about the negative side effects from drugs. Hmmmm....who is funding those pub-lications through advertising dollars? If you guessed pharmaceutical companies, you're right! And with 180,000 Americans dying annually from negative side effects of drugs and interactions with other drugs, it's no wonder the pharmaceutical companies also spend billions annually on lobbyists.

Simple plants that may grow right in your own back yard are often more effective than pharmaceuticals and

rarely have negative side effects. One example is antibiotics. The clients I see who have used three, four or ten
rounds of antibiotics have severely depleted immune systems, making them even more susceptible to the next
virus or bacteria. Instead, if they simply "treat" their cold
or sinus infection with ginger tea and fresh garlic while
getting plenty of rest and at least temporarily eliminating
sugar, they heal faster and strengthen their immune system simultaneously.

If a cold or flu has gone untreated for several days, the
proper combination of antimicrobial herbs (which work
against both viruses and bacteria) will help them feel better within 24 to 48 hours. The first time they use a custom formula, they are amazed at what those simple plants
can accomplish that the expensive antibiotics couldn't.

However, please don't look at herbs as natural drugs
used to provide symptomatic relief alone. For example,
white willow bark tincture is often suggested to ease a
headache, but what is the *cause* of the headache? It may
be a congested liver, hormonal imbalance, the first sign of
a brain tumor or caffeine withdrawal. It's important to
work with a health care practitioner who is a bit of a
detective, always searching for ways to heal the root of the
problem rather than using drugs or herbs as a band-aid.

Mother Nature's plants have an incredible ability to
heal, but at the rate we're taxing our bodies with stress,
poor food choices, a sedentary lifestyle, and excessive
stimulation, we need to learn a healthier way of living
and working. Herbs are a helpful bridge over the river of
a stressful life, offering the promise of long-term wellness.

51. A Guide Through the Health Food Store Maze

In the case of complicated health problems, you're better off with the care and guidance of a trained, professional herbalist. You will usually save money by getting what you need the first time, rather than experimenting with several off-the-shelf products. Working with an herbalist or naturopath who has his or her own dispensary will usually provide you with higher-quality herbs and a personalized formula.

However, if you want to learn a bit about herbs and self-medication for an isolated problem, this guide will help you sort through the overwhelming choices you'll find in the herb section of your local health-food store. There are three basic ways to take herbs, each with advantages and disadvantages.

TEA—The Chinese believe tea is the best way to ingest herbs since you contribute your own healing energy in the process. I agree with this—and know that for the overworked and stressed clients I work with in the West, brewing up a tea to drink (some of which taste nasty) several times a day just won't happen.

However, I love Susun Weed's advice about making a quart of one of the following herbs every day or two: red clover, comfrey leaf, oatstraw or nettles. The benefits are many, but the main advantages are replacing lost minerals which are needed to lessen stress and promote healthy adrenal glands, thereby contributing to greater bone density. Before going to bed, place a couple of hand-fuls (about one ounce) of one of the herbs (or a com-bination) into a glass quart jar, fill with boiled water, cover, and let steep four hours or overnight. Strain the next morning and drink it either hot or iced in the next 24 to 48 hours, with or without honey. Weed says it's even okay to add whiskey as long as you drink the tea! Technically, it's called an infusion when you let a tea steep for several hours, and it's a decoction if it's simmered gently on the stove.

- ◆ ADVANTAGES: Your own "energy" is in the tea since you made it yourself, you increase your consumption of liquids, and it may be less expensive.
- ◆ DISADVANTAGES: It requires drinking quite a lot of tea for therapeutic benefits and can be time-consuming (other than the evening tea recipe above). Also, some antibacterial and antiviral herbs taste nasty; a tincture (described below) requires a dose of only about a teaspoon and tastes no worse than cough syrup.
- ◆ THERAPEUTIC DOSAGE: Drink one to ten cups daily depending on the herb and the illness.

PILLS AND CAPSULES—Sadly, this is the man-ner in which most herbs in this country are consumed. Why? It's easy! We're used to taking pills and now see herbs in capsules as the next quick fix. Choose wisely because herbs prepared in this way are often harvested 12 to 24 months prior to your purchase. Without anything to maintain their potency, you may not get good value; and the pills can be difficult to swallow and digest.

Dried herbs which are properly stored have a shelf life of 12 to 18 months, and optimally should be used as tea or tinctured within 6 to 12 months. Some are best used as fresh plants. When people say "herbs don't work," it's often due to their taking them in pill form and/or not taking the right herb or dose. Frankly, the recommended dosage on the bottle is often minimal; usually it is what your grand-mother can safely take even if she's on several medications.

◆ ADVANTAGES: They're easy; that's it.

◆ DISADVANTAGES: They are of unknown quality and potency; can be hard to swallow and digest; gel caps are contraindicated for some health issues; you don't taste them which can mitigate the affect you want.

◆ THERAPEUTIC DOSAGES: They are difficult to accurately determine since potency is unknown.

Susan's Simple Tip
When buying Chinese herbs in capsule form directly from a licensed acupuncturist, you are much more likely to get a fresh, high quality product than anything off the shelf at the health food store.

TINCTURES—These herbal extracts are made with alcohol and water. They work best for drawing out medicinal properties that are not water soluble. You'll find instructions on how to make them at home in #52. Herbalists often use tinctures because they are concentrated, convenient and easy to swallow. Many contain a greater number of plant constituents than pills or tea because the alcohol and water (called the menstruum) extract more of the whole herb's properties. Tinctures made with fresh plant material are best for some herbs, but most tinctures can also be made using dried plants.

Tinctures make a limited herb supply go a long way. An ounce of dried herb per day is used in medicinal teas; an ounce of dried herb made into a tincture yields ten days of herbal medicine with an adult dose of one teaspoonful three times per day. Tinctures travel well and if a remedy is easier to take, you're more likely to take it consistently. Most herbalists combine two to eight single plant tinctures together for a custom blend. For those who cannot tolerate alcohol, the dose can sit in a teaspoon of hot water for 30 to 60 seconds to evaporate the alcohol. Glycerin tinctures may also be used as an alternative; however, some constituents in certain herbs are not extracted well by glycerin.

- ◆ ADVANTAGES: They travel well, don't freeze, maintain their potency for long periods of time, are easier to swallow than pills or capsules, require a smaller dose than teas for therapeutic purposes, and have greater cost effectiveness for each ounce of dried plant material.

- ◆ DISADVANTAGES: Something other than grain alcohol must be used in the menstruum for those with celiac sprue, a serious gluten allergy. Tinctures may not be suitable for those with alcohol allergies. However, I find that recovering alcoholics do fine by simply evaporating off the alcohol.

- ◆ THERAPEUTIC DOSAGES: Typically one-half to one teaspoon is needed two or three times a day, but it does vary depending on the herb, the person's size, and the health imbalance. Dosages listed on the bottle of mass-marketed tinctures are usually too low to be effective, according to practitioners who have studied in Europe. The reason: the low dose is safer for the manufacturer from a liability point of view.

You will find the best quality tinctures through qualified herbalists. They purchase directly from wholesalers whom they have carefully inspected, or they make their own tinctures using organic herbs when available. If a qualified practitioner is unavailable to you, ask questions about local companies which produce quality herbal tinctures. WhiteDove Herbals and Gaia are two retail brands I trust.

52. Making Your Own Herbal Tinctures

If you're on medications or have a complicated health history, it's best to establish a relationship with an herbalist or other health care provider experienced in the use of herbs. If you expect to be on a particular formula for an extended period of time—for example, with menopause issues—the most economical approach would be for you to make your own tincture. Those experienced in the use of herbal medicine will usually be happy to teach you how to make your own tinctures, but the basics outlined below will help you begin.

Making tinctures at home is easy and far more economical than buying them one ounce at a time at your local health food store. If you start with high-quality herbs and follow these directions, your homemade tincture will be as good as, or better than, anything with a printed label and a much higher price tag. A qualified practitioner will usually be happy to obtain bulk herbs for you to tincture at home, often in one pound quantities which will produce approximately 48 to 64 ounces of tincture.

To make the simplest tincture for home use, fill a clean dry jar halfway with dried herb. Sterilized canning jars work well. Cover the herb with medium-quality brandy, vodka, or rum with a 40 percent or 50 percent alcohol content (80 or 100 proof). Cheap brands contain impurities and unwanted chemicals; expensive brands are unnecessary since the flavor of the herb will dominate in the end. If pure grain alcohol is available, use a mixture of 50 percent water and 50 percent alcohol.

The liquid, called the menstruum, should cover the top of the herbs by about one inch. Cover the jar with a tight-fitting lid. Gently shake the jar so that every bit of the herb is moistened. Label it with the plant name and date—don't rely on your memory.

Herbalists who make their own tinctures use the more exacting method of including a measured amount of both plant material and menstruum. A tincture that is "1:5 50 percent" has one part plant material by weight to five parts menstruum (liquid) which is 50 percent alcohol. There is a wide range of alcohol percentages used, but the method described will work well for home use without complicating your life. When making a tincture from fresh plant material rather than dried, you'll want to use a 1:2 ratio; one part of fresh herb to two parts menstruum. This is due to a high water content in plants before drying.

Ideally, fresh plant tinctures should have 100 percent alcohol for the menstruum with no water added; but if all you have is 150 proof (75 percent alcohol) or 180 proof (90 percent alcohol) grain alcohol, that will work just fine. If this part sounds too complicated, just ignore this paragraph. It describes the methodology of the professional herbalist, not the simplest preparation intended for home use described above.

Leave the jar in a dark, cool place for at least two weeks (four is preferred), shaking it once a day so that the plant material is uniformly wet; otherwise, it won't be fully extracted, yielding a weaker tincture. I prefer letting it macerate, as this procedure is called, for as long as it takes to go through a full cycle of the moon, about four weeks. Depending on the herb you're tincturing, it may require a few more tablespoons of alcohol after the first few days to keep the herb matter covered. Envision your healing intent for this plant each time you shake it: "this will help me build bone density, ease my hot flashes and sleepless nights and balance my blood pressure."

After two to four weeks, it is ready to be poured off, but you can leave it longer when pinched for time. Place several layers of cheesecloth in a wire-mesh strainer with a handle, placing these inside a larger, clean mixing bowl. Pour the liquid and herbs into the cloth and strainer. Gather up the cloth around the wet herb and wring it between your hands. Use a large enough piece of cloth so that the herb doesn't squish out the sides. Squeeze the liquid downward into the bowl. Wear clean dishwashing gloves and clothes you don't care about, as the tincture may stain.

Pour off the liquid tincture into a clean, dry, glass bottle—preferably dark—with a snug-fitting lid, and label it with the date you poured it off and name of the herb. Some sediment may eventually settle on the bottom of the bottle, which is not a problem. But if you like, you can remove the sediment by pouring the clear liquid carefully off the top. This is called decanting. Keep the tincture out of direct light, especially if it's a clear bottle, and store it away from excessive heat.

Due to the alcohol content, a tincture will maintain its potency for many years and will not freeze. In addition to saving money and getting a higher-quality tincture, you're putting your own healing energy into the tincture. What a great way to take charge of your health.

53. Garlic (Allium sativum)—
If I Had to Choose One Herb

If I was stranded on a desert island and could only choose one herb, it would be garlic. Clearly a difficult choice, but garlic has so many uses and can be ingested as a food for many of its medicinal effects. Mince a clove or two each night at dinnertime and swallow with a glass of water to keep your immune system strong. However, if garlic upsets your stomach, start with a very small amount, taken with food, and gradually increase your dose to also help heal that digestive problem simultaneously. Place the minced garlic toward the back of your mouth with a spoon and don't chew it to minimize the odor, which should be gone by the next morning. If you've been searching for a high-return, low-cost way to improve your health, this is it. Don't waste your money on those tablets and pills with the odor removed—the medicinal properties are removed right along with the smell.

Using garlic in cooking is good, too, but the heat breaks down some of the healing properties. Start your recipes by adding a little minced garlic with the olive oil for flavor; then add more raw garlic—without further cooking—for medicinal purposes. You can also make a tincture with it. Because organically grown bulbs contain several times more of the antiseptic substances than those subjected to chemicals, they are my first choice.

One of my favorite uses of garlic is as a vaginal suppository for yeast infections. Starting as soon as you suspect an infection, insert one carefully peeled garlic clove vaginally at bedtime for seven nights. If it doesn't flush out with your urine the next morning, it is as easy to retrieve as a tampon without its string. If you catch the yeast infection early, this is very effective. Even if you're out of town, any market will carry garlic. Drinking lots of water and minimizing sugar in your diet are common sense tips to remember with yeast infections, too.

You'll be amazed at garlic's many medicinal uses:

◆ stimulates digestion and relieves abdominal fullness; helpful for gastroenteritis
◆ chronic or acute candida, thrush
◆ food poisoning
◆ liver congestion (indicated by fatigue first thing in the morning after a good night's sleep)
◆ hypothermia, chills; increases circulation
◆ high or low blood pressure (isn't it amazing it can help *both*?)
◆ congestive heart failure, cardiac asthma, shortness of breath
◆ diabetes (preventative and supportive), hyperglycemia, hypoglycemia
◆ chronic fatigue due to overwork or chronic disease
◆ cold and flu; best if started the first day (one of the best antibacterial, antiviral, antifungal, antiseptic plants available)
◆ digestive and respiratory infections, dysentery, laryngitis, tonsillitis, diphtheria, typhus, cholera

◆ bronchitis, bronchial asthma, lung tuberculosis (TB)
◆ edema, gout, skin rashes
◆ hard deposits: arteriosclerosis, liver cirrhosis, urinary stones
◆ blood clots (thrombosis), phlebitis, varicose veins
◆ high blood cholesterol, triglycerides
◆ tumors, benign or malignant
◆ hay fever
◆ earache, ear infection
◆ intestinal parasites, insect bites

Wow—what a plant! Smaller doses (one-half to one minced clove a day) work well for supporting the immune system, but you'll need two or more minced cloves for its antibacterial and antiviral properties to be effective when you're coming down with something. Up to eight cloves a day may be taken in acute conditions, such as infections. It is one of the most efficient anti-infective and antiseptic remedies available, esteemed worldwide as a super food and super remedy. Garlic's benefits have been well researched, documented and publicized for effectively treating some of the West's most chronic ailments, such as high blood pressure, high cholesterol, arteriosclerosis, diabetes and cancer. However, it is garlic's benefits in both acute and chronic infections of the respiratory, gastrointestinal and epidermal (skin) systems that are recognized as unsurpassed in all the world's medical systems.

Cautions: Contraindicated for premature ejaculation or a tendency to bleed spontaneously. Some say it should not be used during pregnancy or lactation, but many mid-wives say it depends on the person. Garlic may cause flatulence if you have a sensitive stomach, but it can assist with that problem when you build up your dosage slowly and combine it with ginger or peppermint. Those on blood-thinners should have their blood checked regularly and have their medication adjusted as needed. I've worked with a number of physicians to get people off of Coumadin, or at least on a reduced dose—with the help of garlic.

54. Astragalus Root (Huang chi root)— Enhancing the Immune System

For those with chronic immune system problems, including autoimmune diseases, I typically reach for astragalus as part of the appropriate herbal formula. It's also easy to use as a food; the root slices look like tongue depressors and do not modify the taste of soups, sauces or stews. You can even rinse the root off, store it in the refrigerator, and use it again within a couple of days. Your local health food store or co-op will likely carry astragalus root.

Rather than echinacea which I use more for acute infections and the common cold, astragalus is a gentle immune system builder which is perfect for daily use as a tonic for people who seem to catch anything that comes along. Since it's an amphoteric, it actually balances the immune system which makes it helpful with autoimmune disorders. Here are some of the symptoms and illnesses for which you will find astragalus a useful herb:

- exhaustion from overwork or a long illness
- poor endurance and motivation
- frequent or chronic infections
- difficulty keeping weight on
- daytime sweating accompanied by a loose stool
- weakness, low vitality, premature aging
- chronic fatigue syndrome
- AIDS
- allergies

- chronic hepatitis and other liver deficiencies (it's an interferon inducent)
- malnutrition and malabsorption (not absorbing the proper nutrients)
- bleeding (especially uterine bleeding)
- chronic wounds, sores and ulcers
- all infections (including liver and kidney infections, Epstein Barr virus, and HIV)
- cancer of all types
- especially beneficial to the endocrine, immune, digestive, and urinary systems

Caution: Contraindicated in the initial stages of boils and acute infections; best in formula with other herbs for nursing mothers—check with your health care practitioner first.

55. Licorice (Glycirrhiza glabra)— Digestion, Menopause, Adrenal Glands and the Immune System

Currently mislabeled as causing high blood pressure (which it does not), licorice root has been used for centuries with great results. Since it *can* create some water retention around the heart in some people, it does need to be used with caution if you already experience hypertension. Combining it with dandelion leaf, a diuretic, is often enough to alleviate this problem, but you'll be best served by some professional advice in this situation.

Due to its taste, licorice makes a pleasant tea and can also balance some of the more bitter flavors in an herbal tincture formula. Either a tea or tincture of licorice root works well, but the DGL (deglycyrrhizinated licorice) product available at the health food store is not worth your money. When they remove the constituents that may cause trouble for those who have high blood pressure, they remove the majority of medicinal properties, as well.

Some of the many uses for licorice root include:

- ◆ fatigue caused by immune compromise, overwork, stress, adrenal depletion or hormonal imbalance
- ◆ hypoglycemia (low blood sugar)
- ◆ high blood cholesterol
- ◆ PMS
- ◆ menopause symptoms
- ◆ allergic asthma

- allergies in general
- weakened immune system
- dry skin and internal dryness
- coughing due to dryness, irritation or nervousness
- hoarseness, sore throat
- gastric hyperacidity and ulcers
- food poisoning
- urinary irritation and pain due to stones or uric acid
- bacterial and viral infections of the respiratory, digestive, or urogenital systems (including lung TB, pneumonia and hepatitis)
- chronic joint inflammation
- skin problems such as dermatitis, eczema, itching, and cysts
- cancerous tumors

Caution: Contraindicated for those with hypertension or hyperglycemia unless under the care of a qualified practitioner.

56. Hawthorn Berries (Crataegus oxyacantha)—Strengthening and Opening the Heart

Often thought of as *the* remedy for the heart, I also reach for hawthorn often to support women experiencing menopausal symptoms. Not only does it help with hot flashes and irritability, it helps relieve the palpitations which sometimes come with hormone fluctuations. Another common symptom during menopause is indigestion along with heartburn or flatulence—also relieved by hawthorn. And for those of us who have spent most of our lives in our head trying to "figure it all out," hawthorn helps us make the longest journey—from head to heart.

As a heart restorative, it can't be beat. Hawthorn is the perfect herb in a formula for someone with heart disease in their family, or for those who have already experienced a heart attack, high blood pressure, high cholesterol, cardiac edema or hard deposits, such as arteriosclerosis. Nearly all formulas I create have at least one type of berry in them since they are rich in flavanoids. Referred to as "biological response modifiers," flavanoids possess anti-inflammatory, antiallergenic, antiviral and anticarcinogenic properties. I've also witnessed a fabulous response in clients with asthma using a hawthorn tincture on an as-needed basis instead of their inhalers.

Include hawthorn for these conditions:

◆ circulatory problems in general, especially arterial circulation

- high or low blood pressure
- heart disease with angina or peripheral arterial deficiency
- insomnia
- anxiety
- menopause symptoms; hot flashes, irritability, insomnia, palpitations
- cardiac edema, tachycardia, arrhythmia
- hard deposits: coronary sclerosis, atherosclerosis, arteriosclerosis, gallstones, urinary stones
- high blood lipids (high cholesterol)
- digestive enzyme deficiency
- diarrhea
- asthma

Cautions: Due to hawthorn's ability to support the heart, it should be used under the guidance of your health care practitioner if you are on digitalis glycosides, beta blockers or other hypotensive drugs; the dosage of those drugs can often be lessened with the use of this plant.

57. Black Cohosh (Cimicifuga rasemosa/Actaea racemosa)— More than Menopause

Thought of as *the* menopause herb, black cohosh has many other uses. Classified as an adaptogen, it nourishes the adrenal glands which become depleted during times of stress. In simple terms, it helps you adapt to stressful situations. Black cohosh assists with labor when there is a failure to progress and helps mitigate the pain of a difficult labor, but should only be used during the last three weeks of pregnancy. It is known as a "diagnostic agent to differentiate between spurious and true labor pains, the latter being increased, while the former are dissipated under its use," according to John King's *American Dispensary*, 1887. Since black cohosh is also an excellent remedy for neurocardiac syndrome and high blood pressure, it works synergistically in formulation with hawthorn berries.

As a phytoestrogen (plant-based estrogen), black cohosh helps ease excessive hot flashes, delayed or irregular menses, and excessive cramps at the onset of menstruation. But since plant estrogens are living at the time of harvest, nearly all experts agree that black cohosh does not contribute to breast cancer as does synthetic estrogen. This plant is known for easing PMS and irregular menstrual cycles, in addition to helping with:

◆ seizures of all types, including with infants
◆ chronic gastritis
◆ fibromyalgia

- high blood pressure
- cold or flu, if caught early
- PMS with irregular cycles, irritability, anxiety, headache and sleep loss
- amenorrhea (no periods at all, sometimes caused by excessive exercise or anorexia)
- menopause accompanied by hot flashes, dizziness, ringing in ears (tinnitus), palpitations, headaches, irritability
- uterine hemorrhage, mid-month and postpartum bleeding
- asthma
- bronchitis
- high blood pressure
- muscle tension with soreness (including from sprains)
- pain, especially in the reproductive area

Caution: Not to be used during pregnancy, except for three weeks prior to due date, and best avoided during lactation. There is controversy about using it with estrogen-dependant tumors; seek help from your health care practitioner. Caution is also suggested for people with pre-existing cholestasis.

58. *Stinging Nettles (Artica dioica)—Tonic for Restoring Stressed-Out Adrenal Glands and Preventing Osteoporosis*

Typically thought of for allergies of all types, nettles is useful for *much* more. The rich mineral content in nettles (and also red clover, comfrey leaf, oats and raspberry leaf) is a fabulous restorative to the adrenal glands—commonly depleted by stress. It also contains chlorophyll which is a cancer preventative. Used as a tea on a regular basis, this plant restores depleted calcium reserves, thereby helping to prevent osteoporosis. It grows prolifically and is a great cooked green, if you're an adventurous gardener and chef. The stinging aspect of the leaves is eliminated when you cook these mineral-rich leaves. If you buy nettles in pill form at your health food store, look for the freeze-dried version since it captures more of the plant's constituents needed against allergy problems.

Especially good when experiencing chronic and degenerative disorders, nettles has a special affinity for the liver, lungs, intestines, spleen, kidneys, bladder, uterus and connective tissue. This is one plant I suggest as a tea to nearly everyone because it supports stressed-out adrenals without concerns about herb-drug interactions.

To make just under a quart of this nutrient-dense tea, place one ounce in a glass quart-size jar; canning jars are perfect. It should look just a little under half-full with the ounce of dried nettles in it. Add just-boiled water up to the top and cap it snugly before allowing it to steep (sit on the counter) for four hours or up to overnight. The next morning, use a strainer to drain it and squeeze out the remaining liquid before placing the used nettles in your compost or under outdoor plants and bushes for their nourishment. I suggest drinking a quart a day (it replaces a quart of your water consumption) for one to three months, depending on how out-of-balance you feel; then drink one to two cups per day for maintenance.

Consider this nutritive plant to help balance the following:

- ◆ fatigue, especially chronic
- ◆ stress, especially long-term
- ◆ anemia
- ◆ connective tissue weakness (muscle strains and sprains which are slow to heal)
- ◆ scanty breast milk
- ◆ amenorrhea (no period due to excessive exercise or anorexia)
- ◆ PMS
- ◆ menopause symptoms, especially adrenal-related hot flashes
- ◆ hair loss
- ◆ chronic bronchitis, bronchial asthma
- ◆ hay fever, allergic asthma
- ◆ eczema
- ◆ diarrhea, chronic gastric stomach problems
- ◆ urinary infections, acute and chronic
- ◆ burns, bites, stings, wounds
- ◆ skin problems in general

- excess toxins
- urinary stones, gallstones
- edema
- hemorrhoids

Caution: It's a very rare problem, but if you are supposed to limit your calcium intake, be careful since the tea/infusion contains 2,000 milligrams of calcium per quart—this, however, is great news for most of us.

59. Milk Thistle Seed
(Silybum marianum)
Assisting the Over-Taxed Liver

Chinese practitioners consistently place emphasis on the liver—and with good reason. This organ is responsible for flushing all the toxins out of the body. Given the air we breathe, the food we eat and the water we drink, this is a big job. If you toss in pharmaceutical drugs, excess alcohol and smoking you're chances of developing a congested liver go up dramatically. One sign of this condition is never feeling quite refreshed in the morning, even after a good night's sleep. Milk Thistle to the rescue! It promotes bile flow, reducing congestion in the liver and it can help promote healthy bowel movements as well. Since most clients I see suffer from constipation and excess toxins, I reach for this plant a lot. Those with Hepatitis (A, B, or C) or other chronic liver problems would benefit from using milk thistle with the proper guidance.

In addition to restoring the liver, it stimulates circulation, promotes expectoration, benefits the veins and dissolves stones. Nearly all of my clients battling cancer have milk thistle in their formula since they are often undergoing chemotherapy and/or radiation as part of their protocol. Conditions which indicate this plant's use would be beneficial include:

- ◆ liver cirrhosis
- ◆ liver toxicosis and degeneration
- ◆ hepatitis

- low blood pressure
- urinary stones and gallstones
- hemorrhage, especially associated with menstruation
- varicose veins.

Caution: It's best to use this under the guidance of a qualified HCP (health care practitioner) if you have any known sensitivity to plants in the Compositae family. Rare cases of anaphylaxis have been reported.

60. Red Clover (Trifolium pretense)— Calcium and So Much More

Like nettles, red clover contains many beneficial minerals to strengthen bones and replenish adrenal glands which are depleted by stress. It promotes detoxification, dissolves deposits and tumors, reduces inflammation and swelling, and relieves wheezing and coughing. I have personally known several women who were able to avoid a hysterectomy—which their physicians said was their only solution for fibroids—with the use of red clover tincture. For those who struggle with an extreme urgency to urinate, red clover can provide relief. Constipation can be relieved to some degree and it is also helpful against burns and eye inflammations. Its antitumoral properties make it a natural to include in cancer formulas. This herb is particularly well-suited as a tea due to its mineral content and rather pleasant taste, but works well in a tincture, too. Look to red clover for help against the following:

- eczema
- arteriosclerosis
- heavy metal poisoning and drug residues
- tumors, especially of the skin, breasts and ovaries
- gout
- arthritis
- bladder or rectal irritation, including acute bladder infections
- asthma

- coughing, especially spasmodic and whooping cough
- bronchitis
- neurogenic bladder (extreme urgency)
- constipation
- PMS
- wounds, burns, eye inflammations
- insect bites and stings

Caution: None.

61. Dandelion (Taraxacum officinale)— Eases Chronic Constipation, Indigestion and Edema

Next time you see dandelions taking over your yard, do your best to reframe your annoyance. I see this simple plant as the great hope for our Earth; no matter what type of chemicals we use to kill them, they keep coming back. This is a positive sign that our planet can recover from all the crimes we have committed against her. Likewise, dandelion helps our bodies recover from the many poisons we ingest.

Dandelion is an incredible detoxicant. If this simple plant can continually come back after its many assaults, it's no wonder it does an exceptionally good job of expelling toxins. Thankfully, we can expect similar results by using dandelions for our bodies. The best way to use them medicinally is as food. Yes, food. Keep an eye out for dandelion greens at your local health food store. Mostly available in the spring, these mineral-rich greens can be sautéed lightly with a little garlic and olive oil, or tossed with other greens in a salad to mitigate their bitterness.

But when fresh dandelion is unavailable, or you need a larger quantity for medicinal purposes, tinctures and teas work well. Since this simple yet powerful plant is a natural diuretic, it can be combined with licorice root (which can contribute to water retention) whenever there is a concern about high blood pressure. In fact, many of my clients take it to counteract the common pharmaceutical side effect of edema (water retention).

Dandelion root and leaf have slightly different properties. In general, you'll find the same constituents in both, except for the diuretic property which is more prevalent in the leaf. This is a result of its higher potassium content. The root is slightly more helpful as a gentle laxative, but if all you have is the leaf, it can be equally effective in a slightly larger dose. I usually use the leaf since so many of my clients suffer from chronic congestion.

A wonderful ingredient for a daily tonic, dandelion has many uses:

- skin problems such as eczema, acne and herpes I (on the lip)
- arthritis, rheumatism and gout
- liver congestion and detoxification in general
- jaundice, hepatitis
- edema (general, renal and cardiac)
- liver cirrhosis
- arteriosclerosis
- urinary stones
- high blood pressure
- hypoglycemia
- indigestion
- bladder irritation, especially scant and frequent urination
- infections including tonsillitis, mastitis and urinary tract infections
- lymph congestion with swollen glands
- chronic immune deficiency
- connective tissue degeneration (chronic sprain injuries, etc.)

- varicose veins and hemorrhoids
- diabetes (supportive—not a replacement for insulin)
- breast milk insufficiency
- asthma, especially with a cough

Caution: As a gentle tonic, dandelion can be taken for long periods without any side effects, but higher doses of the root tincture may loosen the stool more than desired.

62. White Willow Bark (Salix alba)—
Pain Relief Before Aspirin

When Bayer created aspirin synthetically, they did so by studying Native Americans use of white willow as a pain reliever. However, aspirin has such a low toxic dose that it would not pass the FDA's stringent regulations if approval for it was sought today. Some of the same caution applies to white willow.

Due to its "cooling" nature, willow is effective for many types of infection in addition to its well-known use as a pain reliever. It is also helpful for chronic inflammation which is good news if you're concerned about the side effects of NSAID's (Non-Steroidal Anti-Inflammatory Drugs) like Ibuprofen.

Even though it does not have the broad use of other plants, white willow is so helpful for pain and inflammation, it's a helpful herb to have on hand. Consider using it against the following:

- ◆ headaches and pain in general (but see your health care practitioner to learn about the cause)
- ◆ urinary infections and irritation
- ◆ joint, throat, mouth and eye inflammations from infection
- ◆ nose bleeds, wound hemorrhage
- ◆ chronic diarrhea, dysentery
- ◆ gastric hyperacidity
- ◆ vaginitis (yeast infections)

- slow, painful digestion
- wounds, gangrene
- burns and scalds

Caution: Overdosing may cause internal bleeding. Use with care during pregnancy, when it is best in formulation with other herbs.

63. Siberian Ginseng (Eleutherococcus senticosus)— More Than Just an Energy Herb

Due to its adaptogenic properties (helping you adapt to stress), Siberian ginseng is particularly suited for our hectic and stressful lifestyle in the West. Since it is also indicated for chronic immune problems, endocrine imbalance and ridding the body of excess toxins, it's a perfect ingredient for many formulas.

Not classified as a true ginseng, this herb has many of the same actions as the ginsengs, but at considerably less cost. Some researchers consider it to be superior to the "real" ginsengs. Relatively new on the scene, it was in 1854 that a Soviet botanist identified the plant in the Ussuri region of the Russian Far East. However, it was not identified as an adaptogen until 1958.

Whenever plagued by chronic illness, frequent colds or consistent stress, Siberian ginseng is one of the herbs to consider as a long-term tonic. Like hawthorn, it can help balance both extremes of a problem, such as both hypoglycemia and hyperglycemia which are blood sugar imbalances. This ability to normalize (raise *or* lower something) makes it an amphloteric. Specifically, Siberian ginseng addresses the following:

- ◆ hypothyroidism (insufficient thyroid function)
- ◆ pancreas insufficiency
- ◆ chronic stress or prolonged illness, low energy
- ◆ diabetes (supportive)

- post-surgery healing
- insomnia
- memory and concentration loss
- depression
- poor vision and hearing
- low immunity with chronic infections
- immunodeficiency disorders including AIDS and chronic fatigue syndrome
- anemia
- anorexia
- amenorrhea (loss of periods due to anorexia or excessive exercise) or irregular menstruation
- hypoglycemia and hyperglycemia
- heart palpitations, low blood pressure and moderately high blood pressure
- heart disease, angina
- vascular headaches, dizziness, head trauma
- toxicosis, especially from metals
- inflammation including rheumatoid arthritis
- edema
- chronic bronchitis, coughing
- infections in general, including HIV
- cancerous tumors
- radiation sickness

Caution: Siberian ginseng should not be used when experiencing an acute infection; use with caution (and in combination with other herbs) if you have high blood pressure or any cardiovascular problem. If used as a simple herb—by itself—it's best used in courses; six weeks on and two weeks off.

64. St. John's Wort (Hypericum perfoliatum)—Depression, Wound Healer and Awesome Antiviral

By now you are likely familiar with using St. John's wort against depression. It is often helpful, but as with all illnesses, it's important to work on healing the root cause of the depression. Often it has to do with a congested liver which is frequently overlooked in the West. As with most other herbs, I find it works best in formula with other herbs such as lemon balm, blue vervain and oat seed to balance depression.

St. John's wort is also a terrific antiviral to mitigate the symptoms of genital herpes, shingles, HPV (human papillova virus) which creates genital warts and other viruses which cause colds and flu. Since St. John's wort promotes tissue repair, I often use it for bruises, sprains and strains, especially if a nerve has been damaged. A gentle remedy, St. John's wort is especially well-suited for children and the elderly. It is one of the best plants for treating burns and wounds because it helps heal both soft tissue and damaged nerves. Include it in your formula against the following:

- mild to moderate depression
- bedwetting
- dysmenorrhea (painful, irregular periods)
- urinary stones and pain
- irritable bowel syndrome

- sciatica and spinal pain with a burning sensation or soreness
- headaches, especially migraines
- muscle tension, cramps, spasms, soreness
- bronchitis, especially chronic
- inflammation
- dermatitis
- viral skin conditions such as cold sores (herpes I), shingles and chickenpox
- children's infections (both bacterial and viral)
- animal bites and insect stings
- intestinal parasites (especially in children)
- injury with pain and swelling, including nerve injury
- breast engorgement and lumps
- varicose veins

Cautions: Only use during lactation if under a professional's care. Not intended for use with severe depression. Photosensitivity is possible, as well as gastrointestinal symptoms. Contraindicated with cyclosporine, digoxin, HIV inhibitors, fexofenadine, midazolam, and anticoagulant drugs. Caution is advised for those on low-dose birth control pills.

65. Turmeric (Curcuma longa)— Anti-Inflammatory, Gall Bladder Disease and Cancer

The more I learn about the benefits of turmeric, the more I use this fabulous herb. It's actually the same spice which gives curry that rich golden color, and there are some medicinal benefits from including it in your diet. But to use it therapeutically, a tincture is best.

When I work with a new client who has cancer, I often include turmeric in their formula. Donald Yance, whom I consider to be the leading U.S. expert on integrative medicine and cancer, reports that turmeric is one of the most extensively researched herbs against this life-threatening disease. Since it protects the liver, in addition to being antitumor, turmeric assists in restoring the liver after invasive treatments like chemotherapy and radiation. It also can help prevent cancer.

Several of my clients call it a miracle herb for arthritis pain and other types of inflammation. This is one instance when I prefer to use it as a simple herb (by itself), rather than in formula with other herbs since it is so incredibly effective alone. Those who suffer from inflammation report that it works as well as Vioxx or Celebrex—without the very concerning side effects. Consider using turmeric against these health imbalances:

- cancer of all types
- inflammation including arthritis and rheumatism
- gallbladder disorders

- liver toxicosis and congestion
- hepatitis, jaundice
- high cholesterol
- coronary heart disease
- seizures (including epileptic)
- nosebleeds
- viral infections
- painful digestion, constipation

Caution: Use with caution during pregnancy—best in formulation with other herbs. It is ineffective, and possibly contraindicated, if you've had your gall bladder removed. Professional advice should be sought if you have gallstones or obstruction of the biliary tract. Do not use high doses for longer than two weeks, and avoid excessive sun exposure—like you *always* do, I hope—while using turmeric.

66. Supplements—Keep Them Simple

The whole issue of supplements can get complex and expensive. I infrequently suggest them since I prefer getting necessary vitamins and minerals through quality food and herbal teas. But if you're struggling to make healthier food choices, true whole food supplements can build a helpful bridge. I worry about the temptation to use supplements as an excuse for poor eating habits. If money is tight, you will stretch your dollar much further with the proper food choices than by relying on pills for maintaining health. As I used to say to my then-16-year-old daughter on her way out for the evening, "make wise choices."

Most vitamin and mineral supplements are synthetic and a waste of money, at best. You'll often find unnecessary sugars and fillers present in the cheaper brands. MegaFoods and New Chapter seem pretty good, but tend to be a bit pricey. Usana is a good brand, too, if their multi-level marketing (MLM) set-up doesn't bother you.

Standard Process is a company I think highly of, and they will only sell through qualified practitioners who can make the proper recommendations. Founded by a 1930's Renaissance man named Royal Lee, Standard Process has a very different approach with supplements; they are made of condensed whole foods. And I like the fact that they've stood the test of time. I do offer some of these whole-food supplements to the few clients who don't respond as well to common sense suggestions and herbal support.

But for most of us, the only supplements I recommend are a daily teaspoon of quality cod liver oil (rich in Vitamins A and D) along with nettle tea (#58) and fresh garlic (#53). These are real foods; simple and easy for your body to assimilate. Plus a whole lot less expensive than a handful of pills.

Susan's Simple Tip

I am often approached by people representing MLM companies that offer all types of supplements, fruit juice drinks and the like. I have never carried these products in my dispensary because the few companies that offer a quality product are overpriced and I am not willing to pass on that extra expense to my clients. Buyer beware.

Chapter Five

Special Issues for Women

"Your emotions are your inner guidance system.
Regardless of what supplements you take and what kind
of exercise you do, when all is said and done it is
your attitude, your beliefs, and your daily thought
patterns that have the most profound effect on
your health. You have, within you, the power to create
a life of joy, abundance, and health, or you have the same
ability to create a life filled with stress, fatigue, and disease.
With very few exceptions, the choice is yours."

Christiane Northrup, M.D.
The Wisdom of Menopause

J udy, who was referred to me by a long-term client, was concerned about her recurring yeast infections after taking many rounds of antibiotics. At 36, Judy was slim but hadn't exercised in years and believed the low-fat myth about good nutrition. She noticed her sugar cravings increasing in recent years and found it very difficult to cut back, even after learning from a friend that sugar and white flour products can contribute to yeast infections.

After nearly non-stop infections for three months, Judy and her husband were getting tired of sex being off-limits—not to mention Judy's discomfort—so she sought my help. I knew that changes in her diet were critical for the antifungal herbs to assist her body in healing itself long-term, so I asked her to keep a food diary for two weeks while doing her best to increase quality fats and animal products while eliminating sugar. Writing down her food intake was a great "reality check" on what she truly ate, and helped me find healthy substitutes for her more stubborn cravings.

Within days of being on the right herbal formula (see #71 for more details), Judy felt much better; but I knew it would be temporary if she was unable to change her diet and unable to add moderate exercise to her daily rounds. Thankfully, she found the food changes to be relatively easy after adding more quality fat and protein to her diet, and discovered a bonus—greater energy and less anxiety. I love that type of side effect.

Women are lucky. We have a hard-wired reason to eat well (or at least less) and exercise regularly—beauty. Our attractiveness is often what we get stroked for in this culture, so we have a special incentive to be fit and trim.

Some women are not so lucky; they stay thin without exercising or making conscious food choices. It may sound strange, but I believe these women are unlucky because it's easier for them to make poor health choices. It took years for me to come to this conclusion; I believe I was given a gift when God made me one of the 75 percent of people who get chubby when not eating well and being sedentary.

However, I don't agree with society's penchant for placing our worth squarely on our level of attractiveness— quite the opposite, in fact. But given that that's the way it currently works, I've chosen to see this as a gift. I've also chosen to move from being a high-maintenance woman to a low-maintenance woman, about which you'll discover more in this chapter. Part of being healthy is learning to prioritize all the demands in our lives in ways that work for *us* as women, rather than continuing to accept the roles given to us at birth. Letting go of our superwoman role, releasing our need to control nearly everything around us, and simplifying our relationships are all necessary for us to achieve simple and satisfying health.

This chapter will offer you some of the easiest and least expensive remedies available for everything from yeast infections, to a less than perfect PAP smear, to PMS. One of my most difficult tasks in writing this chapter has been determining where to draw the line since there are so many health issues that women experience. But since there are many good resources on specific health issues (some of which are listed in the Bibliography), I've limited this chapter to the ones you are most likely to experience.

You'll be amazed at some of the uses for garlic—and relieved to know that, in addition to having lots of company when you receive a questionable PAP result (70 percent of all women will at some point), most of those less-than-perfect results will turn around by using simple and inexpensive healing techniques. We may have more health issues, but we are fortunate to live longer than men. I believe part of the reason is because we pay attention to health imbalances before they become crises. Of course, we know how to ask for directions, too.

67. *Superwoman Is Dead*

Well, maybe not dead, but if superwoman keeps going at her current rate, she will at least be dealing with chronic fatigue syndrome, fibromyalgia or very depleted adrenals. And if she's still functioning well physically, I'm betting her family will testify to a serious side effect—chronic bitchiness. When we don't take care of ourselves, everyone around us suffers.

Have you ever noticed that the more gadgets we have to make our lives efficient, the less time we have to nurture ourselves and each other? While there are some modern conveniences—like washing machines—that we may not be willing to eliminate, there are many "technological advances" we can live without.

- Cell phones are handy, but somehow we did muddle through without them just a few short years ago. If you carry one, *choose* when to answer it and for the sake of the rest of us, turn it off in public places. And for everyone's safety, please refrain from chatting while driving.
- Electronic calendars and Blackberries (I call them Crackberries) may streamline life for some users, but most people I know who use one also use a paper version in case they have a crash. Whenever you have to look in two places to know if you're free of appointments, you've just lost your efficiency and complicated your life.

◆ If you have a small business, think carefully about having a website. They take time and money to maintain—not to mention the frustration when they don't work properly—and in some cases do not bring in extra revenue. However, if you need credibility or a way to increase sales, a web site can be the ultimate tool. For help on a bazillion issues for the not-so-technologically inclined, visit *ELance.com*.

◆ For ways to decrease work time and increase personal time, check out my new favorite book: *Four Hour Work Week* by Timothy Ferris. If a website is critical for your business, he will help you minimize what I call the brain damage.

Susan's Simple Tip
This is from the book, *Four Hour Work Week*, cited above. To save time, start checking email and voice mail only at 10:00 A.M. and 4:00 P.M. This one tip has helped me focus more on what is important, rather than getting caught up in other people's urgencies.

These few examples may awaken you to other "modern tools" which create more problems than they solve. Every time you use something considered a modern convenience, take a moment to contemplate whether it saves you time or simply requires storage space, maintenance

costs and cleaning. If you find the benefits do not out-
weigh the costs, take it to a local charity rather than
shoving it toward the back of the closet.

There are lots of ways we create a role for superwomen, many of which have to do with perfectionism.
Many of the superwomen I know can't imagine living in
a house that is vacuumed less than once a day, and their
kids testify that the *way* it is done is important, as well.
Children do need direction if they are to help with tasks,
but when we become so rigid about the specifics it's easy
to say "Oh, never mind. It's easier to do it myself!" Sound
familiar? Not only do we create more work for ourselves
this way, we deny our children the satisfaction of contributing and feeling good about a chore they're able to
complete.

Husbands also report that they give up at helping
around the house after being criticized or instructed
about the nitty-gritty details of their assigned tasks. One
man I know had his wife come home after he had
mopped the kitchen floor, only to have her angrily repeat
the task on hands and knees since that was the only way
she thought it would be clean. A kind husband who
cleans is worth keeping, ladies! Don't criticize him
because he can't live up to your standards. I prefer a house
which is clean enough to be healthy and dirty enough to
be happy.

A significant lifestyle change may be in order if you
are to regain your sanity. Going from a two-income
to one-income household is possible if you're willing to
simplify your life by letting go of some material things.
Two resources for you are *The Tightwad Gazette* by Amy

Dacyczyn and *Your Money Or Your Life* by Joe Dominguez and Vicki Robin; they will help you align your spending decisions with your values. Not only will this allow super-woman to rest, it will also help you spend more time with those you value most. If your "only" accomplishment is raising happy and healthy children, I consider you to be a successful person.

68. Managing PMS Symptoms

Premenstrual syndrome (PMS) has over 150 recognized symptoms, the most common being anxiety, irritability, water retention (including breast tenderness), food cravings, depression, digestive changes, skin problems and a lower pain threshold. Though PMS and painful periods (dysmenorrhea) often go together, they are separate issues.

PMS symptoms vary depending on general health, especially reproductive history. Hormonal balance can be affected by shock, cultural conditioning, family medical history, nutrition and self-image. It's interesting to note that historically, Native American women do not experience PMS. Could it have to do with the belief that their "moon time" was meant for rest and reflection, leaving daily household duties to their male partners during that time?

Nature's design is for menstruating women to rest a few days each month. Sadly, this is not realistic for many; but we do have the ability to slow down a bit during our Moon (period) and take some time for ourselves. Since most of us know about when to expect our Moon, we can plan to do a little less during that time if we make it a priority. Perhaps the reason most us get cramps or lower back pain is to remind us to slow down during our monthly menses. Sacred time alone, defined by each woman, is the best treatment for PMS.

Does the "Inner Bitch" come out due to hormonal fluctuations, or could it be a result of over-doing it?

Women tend to be peacemakers. Most of the month, we smile and get our work done, give praise to others and handle annoyances with some humor and perspective. But pre-Moon, when we have to ask someone to unload the dishwasher every day for three days in a row—only to empty it ourselves later—something can snap!

As always, it's best to seek out a trusted health care practitioner to determine the best protocol for you and your symptoms. But in the meantime, here are some tips for flowing *with* your cycle, rather than struggling against the tide:

- First and foremost, honor this time with a few minutes of rest several times each day during your moon. Turn off the TV and sit quietly next to your favorite picture or looking out the window to appreciate the beauty all around us. Some surroundings (like work) will test your creativity, but you can still find something beautiful, whether it's a bit of green growing between the concrete cracks or the smile on the face of a coworker.

- Repressed anger can lead to headaches, bloating or rage. When you feel it coming on, do your best to find some alone time to scream and yell and swear at the top of your lungs. I have been known to do this sitting in my car two blocks from my home. It's not pretty, but it is effective.

- Herbs may help immediately or they may take one or two cycles to help rebalance your hormones. For PMS symptoms in general, try vitex (also known as chasteberry), skullcap (Scutellaria lateriaflora) and dandelion leaf (Taraxacum officinale). For blood sugar fluctuation and/or fatigue, add Siberian ginseng (Eleutherococcus senticosus) and/or devil's club (Oplopanax horridum). If you're extra stressed, add valerian root (Valeriana officinalis) or passionflower (Passiflora incarnata). If tension headaches are one of your symptoms, add some lavender (Lavendula officianalis) or put a drop of lavender essential oil on each temple. Total dosage for a tincture should be approximately one teaspoon two or three times a day depending on body weight. If you can't get away to the mountains, herbs can bring that mountain refuge to you.

◆ If your PMS symptoms are made worse by painful cramps, add black haw bark (Viburnum prunifolium) and/or cramp bark (Viburnum opulus). If migraines are triggered by PMS, add feverfew (Chrysanthemum parthenium). If skin problems or constipation accompany your symptoms, add yellow dock root (Rumex crispus) and/or chamomile flower (Matricaria recutita). Decreasing your consumption of protein two weeks before your Moon can help, too.

◆ If gas and bloating become worse with PMS, drink some ginger tea or add ginger to your tincture formula. It can also be consumed in the crystallized form which tastes like candy.

◆ Good nutrition, as always, often provides improvement. Cutting back on sugar is helpful for all of us, but especially if you suffer from PMS. If that sounds totally unrealistic just before your Moon, do the best you can the rest of the month and you'll soon find the cravings lessen. Try a drop or two of gymnema tincture (an Ayervedic herb) on the tongue which will make sweet things taste nasty—it works amazingly well. When you really want a sweet treat, enjoy a teaspoon of raw honey.

◆ Decrease your use of nicotine, caffeine and table salt, as well. Sea salt is fine.

◆ If skin problems accompany PMS, reduce your intake of animal fats and calcium supplements, emphasizing vegetable proteins (beans, fermented soy, etc.) and greens which are a good calcium source.

69. *Breast Cancer Prevention*

Breast cancer is the disease most women fear more than any other, but note the following statistical contrast to keep this in perspective: one in 30 women will die of breast cancer while *one in two* die of heart disease. Since CHD (Coronary Heart Disease) is also the number one killer of men in the U.S.—and the guys will most likely only read that chapter—I included the information on heart support under #84. Please read that section for yourself, since CHD is statistically more likely to kill you than breast cancer.

The percentage of women dying from breast cancer has remained virtually unchanged since the 1950's until 2002. For the past six years, we have seen the first decrease in breast cancer since statistics have been monitored. This drop is strongly correlated with hundreds of thousands of women ceasing use of HRT (hormone replacement therapy) when we were informed about further side effects of these hormonal drugs. A study released in December, 2006 showed a drop of 7% since the media published the connection between HRT use and breast cancer. If you can manage your menopausal symptoms without HRT, it's clearly best to do so.

Based on both research and empirical evidence, I am convinced that the majority of breast cancers are causally related to the high levels of radiation and chemicals in our air, water, soil and food. U.S. government researchers estimate that 80 percent of all cancers are environmentally linked. Many studies reveal that 80 to 90 percent of

all cancer is preventable. See the World Health Organization online, specifically *Who.int/cancer/prevention.org*.
But beware: many websites tout "cancer prevention" but
are actually promoting early detection which, once again,
is often about the drug companies and medical device
companies making money.

When did you last hear about raising money to *prevent*
cancer? Probably never. Preventing cancer through
lifestyle choices is not glamorous and doesn't produce
direct profits for corporate America since the techniques
are so simple and cheap. Charging to the rescue to *treat*
cancer gets all the attention because pharmaceutical companies and others have so much to gain financially.

Warning: be aware that early detection can often lead to
over treatment of the disease using chemotherapy, radiation and surgery. Donald Yance's book, *Herbal Medicine,
Healing and Cancer* can help you and your health care
practitioner determine when better nutrition and improved lifestyle choices are more likely to be effective
without damaging side effects. Many of the clients I work
with who have cancer are experiencing secondary cancers,
mostly in the liver and bones, due in part to medical treatment they received the first time they were diagnosed.

I'm on a personal crusade to get the word out about
true cancer prevention; preventing breast cancer isn't as
simple as an annual mammogram which is still only early
detection, not prevention. To prevent breast cancer we
need to take individual and collective action. Science
does not validate all of the following prevention methods
because the money for scientific research is poured into

the money-makers: early detection and treatment. But lifestyle choices are major factors not only with breast cancer and cancers of other types, but to all potentially lethal diseases.

Susan's Simple Tip

Mammograms are a valid concern to many women; not only because of the radiation exposure, but also due to the theory that you might increase cancer activity with a mammogram if cancer is present. There is a better solution. Ultrasound, also called sonography, is an imaging technique in which high-frequency sound waves that cannot be heard by humans are bounced off tissues and internal organs. Their echoes produce a picture called a sonogram that is an equivalent diagnostic tool, compared to mammography. Ask your doctor; we currently have too few clinics offering this option.

The following is a brief overview of the simplest and most effective ways to reduce your chances of getting breast cancer. Much of this information was derived from Susun Weed's awesome book, *Breast Cancer? Breast Health!*, a highly recommended read. All of her books are excellent resources. The following will help protect you:

Reproductive Factors

◆ Giving birth after the age of 20 and nursing the baby for at least three months. Nursing longer than three months decreases your chances even further.

◆ Maintaining regular menstrual cycles at 25 to 30 day intervals, except during premenopause.

◆ Avoiding synthetic estrogens of all types including birth control pills, and especially, hormone replacement therapy (HRT). Eight percent of all breast cancers are attributed to their use; realistically, that number is probably much higher.

Lifestyle Factors

◆ Keeping your weight within 10-20 pounds of your ideal range. Postmenopausal women who are 50 pounds or more overweight are one-and-a-half times more likely to develop breast cancer.

◆ Exercising regularly. Women who are physically active and eat a cancer-preventing diet lower their risk, no matter how much they weigh. One study suggests that exercising two and a half hours weekly reduces your chance of contracting breast cancer by 40 percent, and three and a half hours weekly reduces your risk by 70 percent. Get after it, girls!

◆ Avoiding organochlorines which are chlorine-based chemicals. Herbicides, pesticides, chlorine bleach, most disinfectants, and many plastics contain these dangerous chemicals. To avoid these harmful chemicals buy only organic butter, dairy, grains, beans and meats. Use glass for food storage rather than plastic, don't drink chlorinated water and avoid showering in chlorinated water.

◆ Avoiding the microwave, especially for actual cooking. Little hard evidence exists since no one has a dollar to make from learning the truth, but I became convinced when I read a study which involved sprouting seeds. When the seeds were watered with microwaved water they refused to sprout! That's enough evidence for me—plus some uncommon sense.

Dietary Factors

◆ Some research attributes as much as 25 percent of all breast cancers to dietary fat, but that's not the real story. The women of Crete receive 50 percent of their calories from fat, yet have the lowest incidence of breast cancer in the world. It's the *quality* of the fat and whether it's part of a calorie-balanced diet (maintaining your weight) that makes the difference. Avoid all hydrogenated oils, margarine, and vegetable oils. Instead, choose quality olive oil and organic butter. Olive oil, packed in a can to protect it from light, is the least costly of the two.

◆ Eat an abundance (five to seven servings) of fruits and vegetables; studies show that those who do, have up to 50 percent less chance of getting cancer than the average American who consumes one to two servings a day—if you count orange juice, which I don't. Organic produce is best, but if it's not available, don't stress about it. Using a drop of soap with a vegetable brush is a reasonable second choice; I still believe the good in the broccoli outweighs the chemicals they may have put on it.

◆ Foods from the bean family, including red clover blossoms, lentils and soy beans can decrease breast cancer risk. Legumes contain enzymes which reduce the production of estradiol and plant hormones which keep estradiol out of breast cells.

◆ Some studies suggest that daily consumption of red meat increases your cancer risk, but they make no distinction between commercial beef and that which is raised without hormones (i.e. synthetic estrogens) or antibiotics. Small amounts (the size of a deck of cards) of red meat two to four times a week offer optimum nutrition when you choose organic meats. Grass-fed beef and buffalo is best and the most expensive— countered easily by consuming smaller amounts in healthy balance with other foods.

◆ Studies available through *webmd.com* indicate that women whose diets were high in fiber had 20 to 30 percent less incidence of breast cancer than those with fiber-poor diets. Eat your whole grains, beans, fruits, and vegetables regularly.

Health Care Factors

◆ Regular use of many prescription drugs can increase your risk of breast cancer. Beta blockers treat high blood pressure, but suppress production of anticancer melatonin. Prozac and Elavil, both anti-depressants, promote the growth of cancer which has already started to grow. Long-term use of steroids and cortisones increase cancer risk, too. There are safe and effective alternatives for nearly any condition treated by prescription drugs. Seek the help of a qualified herbalist or naturopath.

◆ Chronic viral infections increase breast cancer risk. Even a chronic bacterial infection can weaken the immune system, which indirectly increases breast cancer risk. Donnie Yance, a talented herbalist who works with many women diagnosed with breast cancer, believes that having a genetic predisposition to a weak immune system is a very strong risk factor.

◆ According to Susun Weed, author of *Breast Cancer? Breast Health!*, regular use of screening mammograms are dangerous for premenopausal women. For postmenopausal women, they can increase the time between the detection of cancer and death (from any cause), but they don't reduce the actual risk of cancer—nor do they prevent it. Monthly self-examination of your breasts provides early detection at lower cost, without the danger of yearly screening mammograms. According to one English study, women find their own breast cancers 90 percent of the time. Take this a step further by asking your partner for a "breast massage" at least once a month, rather than looking for cancer. Or if it makes you feel better, schedule a mammogram— or preferably an ultrasound—after discussing it with your health care practitioner. *You* are in charge of your body.

70. *From High Maintenance to Low Maintenance*

As women, we are acutely aware of the pressure on us to look good. Historically, women in our culture have been valued mostly for their appearance, which doesn't say much for our evolution. I enjoy looking attractive as much as the next gal, but in the interest of mental health and creating more time for myself and what is most important to me, I have slowly modified my "getting ready" routine in the direction of lower maintenance.

Becoming a low-maintenance woman will save you time and money, and sends a valuable message to any young woman in your life. Most adults live by the adage "do as I say, not as I do"; however, I believe that the best sermon is a good example. Be that example by minimizing the hours, energy and financial resources you invest in looking your best.

In addition to personal hygiene modifications, you can become more low-maintenance by rolling with the punches in life. Women have so many to-do's on their plates, it's easy to become obsessed with having everything go according to plan. Since that is rarely the way life works, planning in pencil helps us to flow *with* the river of life, rather than constantly paddling upstream.

I use a mechanical pencil now rather than a pen to write down appointments in my day planner. Clients need to change their appointments for a multitude of reasons: a child becomes ill, a flat tire greets you as you enter

the garage in the morning—and these are the easy things!
We become high maintenance to others when we yell
over things we have absolutely no control over. Once
you start to lose it, do your level best to breathe deeply.
One full breath can calm you instantly, helping you see
creative options that were clouded by rage.

Try some of the following ideas to decrease the resources you spend on general life maintenance:

◆ Find a five-minute hairstyle that looks great.
   Your hair stylist can make recommendations
   for your hair type, facial shape and lifestyle.
   I have been thrilled with the ease this creates
   in my life.

◆ Simplify your wardrobe. Most women gravitate
   toward their favorite colors, but if you're at a loss
   as to which ones look best on you, consult a
   trusted friend or professional. Once you have
   identified the one or two colors which look best
   on you, get rid of everything (well, almost
   everything) which does not coordinate with
   those basics. I wear black a lot, especially
   when traveling, because it looks great with
   nearly everything, is flattering to the figure and
   rarely shows soil. Bright colors complement
   black well and give me the spice I like in
   my look.

◆ Simplify your accessories. Once you've identified
   the clothes that work best for you, work on
   paring down your accessories, as well. A few

classic pieces can look great with many outfits
and sticking with either gold or silver helps
simplify your jewelry.

◆ Create an everyday make-up routine you can
accomplish in five minutes. It can be done
and will allow you more time for the important
tasks. Consult a down-to-earth cosmetics
consultant if you need some assistance, telling
her upfront about your goals. I hope one goal
will be to use skin care items you would be
willing to eat—because you are, essentially,
through your skin, the body's largest organ.
See Susan's Simple Tip following these bullets
for a skin care idea.

◆ Re-think the whole manicure thing. One of the
most time-consuming aspects of the dress-for-
success mode of the 1980's was the highly
polished, brightly colored, acrylic nails craze.
This may be the most time-consuming of all your
maintenance issues. At the very least, get rid of
the fake nails since they prevent your natural
nails from growing and breathing properly.
Those fumes are unhealthy for all of us. Also,
check Appendix A for information on nail spas
potentially being one of the places to pick up
bacteria that don't respond to antibiotics. There
is a simple beauty in neatly filed, unpainted,
buffed nails.

◆ Kick off your high heels. Any podiatrist will tell
you that women who regularly wear high heels

suffer from bunions and calluses on their feet—
plus calf, knee and back problems. Yes, many
men find high heels sexy; but if you're still
wearing them daily for that reason, it's time for a
shift in your social circle.

Susan's Simple Tip

My physician and friend, Jacqueline Fields, M.D.,
has created a skin care line I think is terrific; for
more information, call The Healing Gardens at
970-472-6802 for a catalog. And no, I'm not
getting any kick-backs.

71. *Stop Carrying a Purse Large Enough to be a Weapon*

When I see a yoga student with one shoulder clearly higher than the other, I can usually predict how she carries her purse. You might think that the shoulder with the purse is lower, but it's actually higher due to our subconscious efforts to keep it from sliding off. A purse is just like your income: however large it is, you'll find a way to push it to the limit. So to start, vary which shoulder you hang it from—on the left going into the store and on your right coming back to the car.

To reduce the weight, start by choosing the right bag—assuming you can't get by with putting your lipstick and a bit of cash in your pockets. Something to carry credit cards, cash and lip color doesn't need to be very big. Any other items you think you can't live without can usually be kept in the glove compartment of your car or stowed in your desk drawer at the office.

When traveling, I suggest a small back pack to evenly distribute the weight since you will likely add a book, bottle of water, fresh or dried fruit and your passport to your short list of "must-haves." Another good option is a small fanny pack.

If you've never experienced the freedom of not having to lug around a huge purse full of heavy items you don't need and rarely use, now is a good time to start. Many structural imbalances can be caused by a heavy purse carried consistently on the same shoulder.

72. Yeast Infections

Yeasts are common in our environment; living in soil, on fruits and vegetables, and thriving wherever there is decay. One type of yeast, Candida albicans, is chronic and systemic so you may need to consult a practitioner for help. Candida was the trendy "disease" of the nineties and often over-diagnosed; but there are many legitimate cases of candida becoming out of balance throughout the body. When in doubt, seek the care of your health care practitioner.

What I can address here are generic yeast infections, often caused by the use of antibiotics (especially broad spectrum) and/or too much sugar in the diet. Your basic vaginal infection (also known as bacterial vaginosis) is often triggered by antibiotics which strip away the healthy microflora in the intestines along with the bacteria they are trying to kill. This sets up a pH imbalance which gets worse when you consume sugar and/or foods which quickly convert to sugar, such as processed flours in crackers, cookies, tortillas and breads.

These refined carbohydrates (including soft drinks) contribute to recurring yeast infections, but hormonal levels can affect the growth of yeast, too. During pregnancy and with the use of the contraceptive pill, a woman is more likely to suffer from yeast overgrowth. The use of douches as a means of personal hygiene may contribute to yeast overgrowth because the beneficial bacteria are washed away, shifting the vaginal pH. Symptoms can be many and varied, but for most women, they include vaginal discharge (think cottage cheese) and itching, often accompanied by redness of the labia.

Vaginal Suppositories

When caught early, my favorite remedy for yeast infections is garlic. Carefully peel a clove of fresh garlic without nicking it. Insert it vaginally just before bedtime and the clove will likely be released automatically the next morning when you go to the bathroom. If not, it is no more difficult to reach than a tampon which lost its string, and should be removed after you get up. Continue inserting one garlic clove nightly for seven to eight nights and it will likely take care of your infection if you catch it in the "Do I have a yeast infection?" stage.

If the infection is more firmly established, make up some boric acid capsules to use in a similar fashion for seven to ten days. Boric acid is easily purchased at your local pharmacy, along with either 00 or 000 size gel caps (ask your pharmacist). Shake out some of the boric acid onto a clean plate or the inside of the lid. After separating a gel cap, simply scoop up the boric acid into the long end of the gel cap and place the top back on it. This remedy was given me by a family physician many years ago and is very effective.

Nutrition

If this is not your first yeast infection, take a careful look at your diet. Most of us consume too much sugar and other refined carbohydrates. Eliminate—or at least significantly limit—all sugar and most fruits while you're healing. Sugars include honey, molasses, maple syrup, and any food with sugar added to them. Acceptable fruits include papaya, pineapple and pears. Also eliminate alcohol and refined carbohydrates such as white bread and pasta, cakes, cookies, pastries and sauces thickened with flour.

- ◆ Because dairy products (milk, cheese, butter) are transformed into sugars by digestion that feed the infection, eliminate them, too.
- ◆ Limit unrefined carbs until after your infection has cleared.
- ◆ Eat plenty of fresh veggies, beans, tofu, seeds, nuts, and plain, whole (not low-fat) "live" yogurt
- ◆ Drink four quarts a day of water and herbal teas; no coffee, fruit juice or soft drinks.

Supplements

The longer I'm in practice, the less I suggest supplements. For the most part, I feel strongly that we should work hard to get our vitamins and minerals from the foods we eat. For the occasional yeast infection, you should not need additional supplements; but if you're struggling with this issue on a regular basis, the following can help (in order of importance):

- ◆ one clove of minced raw garlic (save your money—don't buy the "odor free" capsules)
- ◆ acidopholus/bifidus (two grams powder three times a day between meals)
- ◆ vitamin C (500-1,000 mg twice a day)
- ◆ B-complex (50-100 mg twice a day)
- ◆ beta carotene (25,000 IU twice a day)

- caprylic acid (as directed on label)
- vitamin E (400-800 IU a day)

Helpful Herbs

As always, a custom blend that takes into account your constitution and other health problems is best. If you have no allergies and are on no medications, the following herbs can help fight a yeast infection from the inside: calendula, lemon balm, burdock root, black walnut hull, marigold, and pau d'arco.

73. Bladder Infections

Otherwise known as UTI's (urinary tract infections), these bothersome infections are more than an annoyance. Repeated infections stress your immune system and indicate a need for change in your daily habits. They are often the result of stress, limited consumption of water, inadequately-treated vaginal/yeast infections, using "feminine hygiene products," overdouching, poor nutrition or some type of unfriendly bacteria which has made its way into the urinary tract. Less common causes of chronic UTI's include kidney stones and structural blockages.

Some parts of the body, such as the bloodstream, are alkaline under healthy condition; other places prefer to be acidic—two examples are the vagina and urinary tract. An acid pH keeps out microbes that would grow in these locations if they were alkaline. These normally acidic areas can become alkaline when you are stressed, or when acid-secreting friendly bacteria are wiped out by antibiotics. Ironically, antibiotics are usually suggested by modern medicine which can set up the cycle again with another yeast infection, which may lead to another bladder infection!

Helpful Herbs

- ◆ Bearberry (Arctostaphylos uva-ursi), is a classic for UTI's and very effective in a formula with other herbs. It is usually prescribed in tea form in order to increase consumption of liquids which is critical.
- ◆ Marshmallow root (Althaea officinalis) is very soothing due to its mucilaginous or moistening

properties, but don't be surprised if it looks
rather thick and viscous in tincture form—this is
what makes it so healing.

◆ Yarrow (Achillea millefolium) is a fabulous
hemostatic which means it helps stop bleeding;
so it's a good choice when there is some blood in
the urine accompanying your infection. Pay
special attention to all recommendations when
blood is present as that sometimes indicates a
more advanced infection.

◆ Comfrey leaf (Symphytum officinalis) was
recently maligned as being toxic which is
completely untrue as long as you use the leaf.
Using the root for extended periods has been
shown to create some toxicity when used alone.
Think of comfort when you see comfrey; it's very
soothing to the internal tissues, including those
lining the urinary tract. Comfrey leaf also
reduces inflammation and pain.

◆ Cornsilk (Zea mays) helps to "clear heat,"
thereby reducing infection and inflammation,
and also helps to stop unnatural discharges. It is
also helpful in resolving urinary stones and
reducing bladder irritation or pain. It's very
gentle with no contraindications.

Nutrition

◆ You may want to consider a three-day fast,
consuming only bone broths to give your body
the energy it needs to heal the infection.

◆ Avoid sugar and refined products, including alcohol and carbonated beverages.

◆ Whole foods, especially vegetables, will assist in healing after the first two to three days, but avoid citrus fruits.

◆ Celery, parsley and watermelon act as natural diuretics and cleansers.

◆ Unsweetened cranberry juice is extremely beneficial, but too tart to drink at full strength. Mix four ounces of it with 20-30 ounces of water to make "cranberry water," a helpful dietary addition if UTI's are a common problem.

74. The Bad PAP (Cervical Dysplasia)

Dysplasia (having abnormal cells on the cervix) is not the same as having cancer. A lot of panic results from common misunderstandings about this part of a woman's body. Inflammation of the cervix is called cervicitis, a term often lumped together with dysplasia and other non-malignant cell changes on the surface of the cervix. Hyperplasia is a term that means the cells are growing a bit too fast and too thick, perhaps in response to repeated irritation. New cells born into this stressed tissue are not always healthy, especially if nutrition and/or hormonal imbalances are present. And stress can slow the body's ability to self-repair.

A common condition strongly associated with dysplasia and cervical cancer is human papilloma virus, known as HPV, which is responsible for genital warts. Contrary to popular belief, contracting this sexually-transmitted infection is not a certain path to cancer. See my notes below for managing this without invasive treatments.

There's a new HPV vaccine called Gardasil that's widely touted today. I have serious concerns about it. In addition to the fact that we are using our young girls as guinea pigs during or before puberty, Christiane Northrup, M.D. stated on the Oprah show in 2008 that only four strains of the over 100 known strains of HPV out there lead to cervical cancer, and the death rate for that type of cancer is decreasing each year. She recommends, as I do, to forget Gardasil and increase immune response through diet and exercise instead—plus educate your daughters and granddaughters about sexual choices. Northrup also states that those four strains of HPV that can lead to cervical cancer only do so when the body's immune system is already compromised.

I find the National Vaccine Information Center at *nvic.org* to be a great resource for data on this issue. They report that as of August 2007, 2,207 adverse reactions to Gardasil had been reported. Among those reactions:

◆ five girls died
◆ 31 were considered to be in a life-threatened state
◆ 1,385 required a visit to the emergency room
◆ 451 of the girls have not recovered
◆ 51 of the girls were disabled

All of these side effects for a vaccine that *might* prevent a few strains of HPV, an infection that clears up on its own 90 percent of the time, according to Dr. Northrup. I'm confident the numbers of adverse reactions are significantly higher by now, after the media frenzy accompanying the release of Gardasil.

Helpful Herbs

This is one situation where I highly recommend working with your health care practitioner for a more personalized approach. If he or she is uneducated in forms of treatment other than invasive cryogenic freezing or harsh drugs, arm yourself first by reading the appropriate section of *Herbal Remedies for Women* by Amanda McQuade Crawford before your appointment.

The most important herbs against cervical dysplasia are astringents with an affinity for the reproductive tissues, astringents such as periwinkle leaf (Vinca major) and antimicrobial vulneraries such as calendula (Calendula officinalis L.) or goldenseal (Hydryastis canadensis)—but a customized formula is needed. I've found it helpful to simultaneously use a vaginal treatment consisting of natural sponges soaked in a combination of essential oils, including tea tree and thuja, which are suspended in a carrier oil (like olive oil) to minimize harshness. Please see *Herbal Remedies for Women* (in Bibliography) for specifics. It is a fabulous resource.

Nutrition

Avoid excess alcohol, caffeine, fried foods, dairy, oats, bread, hot spices, pungent foods (like pickles and pre-served meats), preservatives, sugars and any additives. Include plenty of cleansing raw foods: vegetables juices, fresh fruits and vegetables, brown rice and quality protein.

Lifestyle Choices

Because stress can make this, and many other conditions, worse, this may be the perfect time to add yoga and/or meditation to your daily routine. Consider getting coun-seling, especially around any lingering issues regarding sexuality. Without even improving their diet or taking herbs, women with severe cervical cell changes who med-itated for 20 minutes a day for eight weeks, were found to have a cervix on the mend upon retesting. Most of the time, you have some time to try these non-invasive meth-ods without fear of developing cancer—but always talk to your health care practitioner first.

75. Pregnancy and Preventing It

Even though there may be little to fear by being on birth control pills (BCPs) for a few years while managing and/or preventing pregnancies in your twenties, I am not a fan of any pharmaceutical dictating our monthly cycles. Especially if you've been on BCP's for several years, or are moving into your mid-thirties, it's time to search for a better alternative.

Using an old-fashioned diaphragm can offer very good pregnancy protection when used properly; and after learning that most of the women who work at Planned Parenthood use IUDs, I did some research to discover they have come a long way since the seventies when we worried about them puncturing the uterine wall or causing a life-threatening infection. But if you are not through bearing children, I highly recommend the following simple approach outlined in Toni Weschler's *Taking Charge of Your Fertility*.

Through the use of a daily temperature chart and checking your cervical fluid for thickening (which indicates fertility), Weschler does a great job helping us to either achieve or prevent pregnancy, but with an added bonus: you also get to know your body a lot better, which will serve you well for decades. From early detection of certain cancers to sensing a hormonal shift when entering premenopause, having an intimate and knowledgeable relationship with your body serves you well psychologically and physically.

According to the American Society of Reproductive Medicine, infertility affects men and women equally in the United States; about 10 percent of those who were of reproductive age in 1997 were affected. At the beginning of Chapter Three on Lifestyle Issues, I shared the story of Sandra who came to see me about fertility issues. She is a great example of how the smallest shift can result in a healthy baby nine months later. But, most of the people I see about fertility issues need to start with their diet.

I've previously mentioned the Weston Price Foundation (*WestonAPrice.org*) as a great nutritional resource. The original work of this U.S. dentist in the 1920's and 30's clearly demonstrated the connection between nutrition and fertility. Every group of native people he studied around the world had virtually no issues with fertility (or dental decay or heart disease or cancer) until they adopted a Western diet of refined carbohydrates and sugar. Then it only took one generation for all of our Western diseases to show up, including fertility problems.

Step one to having a happy, healthy baby is to create a happy, healthy body for yourself. In addition to whole food choices, moderate exercise can help you take a pregnancy to term. Sometimes, I have to encourage a woman to reduce exercise since training for triathlons and the like can easily reduce fertility—even to the point of temporarily stopping the monthly cycles altogether. Once food and exercise choices are in alignment with health, drinking a daily quart of a strong infusion (tea) of red clover will often be enough to achieve and maintain a pregnancy. Occasionally, a natural progesterone cream will need to be used if miscarriages are an issue.

Once you're certain that you've populated the planet properly, I highly recommend that your male partner obtain a vasectomy. A respected mentor of mine suggests this may interfere with a man's chi—which is entirely possible—but after decades of dealing with monthly cycles and bleeding, hormonal shifts, pregnancies, nursing, possible abortions and then menopause symptoms, I think we women have done enough. Targeting a future date, after which there will be no more sex, is often necessary for compliance. Tell him to just get over it.

76. Magnificent Menopause

What will really be magnificent is if I can get you started down the road of hormone shifts in a 500-word tip. Even though a personalized approach works best, depending on your symptoms and other health issues, most women will see major improvements after two to four weeks by making the following life improvements:

◆ Clean up your diet following the tips in Chapter One; especially important is getting enough quality fat to reduce sugar cravings and nourish you from the inside out.

◆ Move (exercise!) that widening bum on a near-daily basis following the tips in Chapter Two.

◆ Drink a quart a day of nettle tea (#58) as a great start to nourishing your adrenal glands, which can help relieve hot flashes, insomnia and early signs of arthritis.

◆ Cut something out—preferably part of your work week. It's time for YOU now; taking time to rest and get creative will help ease many menopausal symptoms. If you have thyroid problems, it may be time for indulgent bed rest.

◆ Take Susun Weed's advice in *The New Menopausal Years*—at the first sign of symptoms, do nothing. That's right, nothing. Westerners are very quick to pop a pill or sign up for surgery when less-invasive choices would actually work better without the negative side effects. Sit,

breathe, pray and ask for guidance—perhaps
from those a little older and more experienced.
Then start collecting information and
researching your options.

If you're already taking good care of yourself with
nourishing whole foods, regular body movement and a
stable of supportive friends, you'll find this natural transition to be much gentler. Many native women experience no or few menopausal symptoms. The whirlwind life
many of us lead in the West contributes greatly to
unpleasant hormonal shifts. Menopause is a great time to
take stock of whether all those forms of technology truly
provide assistance in your life or provide more insanity.

As is evident by Christiane Northrup's *Wisdom of
Menopause*, there are some fabulous resources available about a subject that was nearly taboo 20 years
ago. Use those resources and make this time an exciting
transition—to the point when you do what you please
without worrying what others think. I'm turning 50 the
month before this book is published, and I love this
time! This is when we get to embrace one of my favorite
quotes by Eleanor Roosevelt, "What other people think
of me is none of my business."

77. Cosmetic Surgeries

I fully acknowledge that this tip may make you hate me, but I am nothing if not direct and honest. Naturally, I want you to feel good about your body; for some of us, making our physical appearance look as good as possible helps us enjoy being in our bodies. It's a good thing to want to look better when it leads us to better food choices, moving our bodies, changing our 25-year-old hairstyle and getting rid of unworn clothes.

With that said, allow me to lovingly express something to all those who have already "had some work done" and are contemplating more, as well as those who may be considering cosmetic surgery for the first time. Investing in a few hours of therapy might help you feel just as good about yourself as spending way more money on surgery—and risking death. See Appendix A on drug-resistant bacteria before scheduling an appointment with your surgeon.

Is it a bad thing to grow older? Is it a bad thing to have lines on our faces and a droop in our boobs or bum? Read #78 on Letting Go to put things into perspective and then consider this: every woman I've worked with in the past 12 years who has had breast augmentation tells me two things. First, her surgeon made her breasts larger than she wanted and larger than she requested. What the hell is that about? And second, they all tell me they wish they hadn't had it done.

Perhaps I work with a select group of women who decided after-the-fact that future surgeries every 10 to 15 years just to keep "the girls" up there just wasn't worth the pain, hard breasts, lack of nipple sensitivity, expense or possible elevated risk of breast cancer. Most of the women I know who have had breast augmentations are not even told they will likely need to be "re-done" in the future; I consider this to be malpractice. You should know about all potential side effects, including the expense and pain of going through this surgery again...and again.

It may be easy for me to pass judgment since my smaller-than-average breasts are still pretty perky as I approach 50, but after losing a dear friend to a superbug infection she caught in the hospital during "routine surgery," I want you to make a conscious choice regarding elective surgery. Is it worth possibly dying in order to have a "better" body?

Susan's Simple Tip

How 'bout a simpler and less invasive way to improve your body's appearance? I'll give you three. First, practice yoga and instantly "lose" 10 pounds visually with an improved posture. Second, lift weights for strong pectoral muscles under your breasts—I think this is partly why mine are still fairly far North of my belly button. Third, to erase those little lines above your lip—smile!

78. *Letting Go*

It's 5:30 P.M. on Friday, February 29, 2008 and I've just returned from a matinee movie. On the way to the theater to spend 96 minutes and $5.50 on a movie I knew little about, *Juno*, I felt guilty for playing instead of working on the final edit for this manuscript. Although I had no serious deadline, I had worked on it passionately all week, and was also giving a presentation to the Wonders of Women conference on Saturday, a day I normally don't work.

Can you see my workaholism here? I still felt guilty about going to a movie, even though I'd been working like a fiend all week. Ladies and gentleman, this is bullshit! Pure and simple bullshit!

The good news is, on the brief drive to the movie theater, I embraced the guilt, had a chat with myself about my week's productivity, and let go of it. *What* did I have to feel guilty about? I decided that being in the presence of a good piece of creative work (which *Juno* was) would fuel my own writing creativity. And, it did! Now it feels good to write, instead of a few hours ago, when my creativity became stagnant and I needed to stop and go to a movie.

Now, I only have 30 minutes left to write before a friend comes by for dinner after a day of skiing. But it's still 30 minutes and I really *want* to work on my writing, rather than feeling blocked and unimaginative. It's ironic that my next tip to write about is letting go. It seems paradoxical that I'm writing about that, given that I'm a recovering control freak and workaholic. Really. Just ask my sister; she'll vouch for the control freak part. My daughter will vouch for the recovering part. Thank God.

One of my favorite phrases is, "Everything I've let go of has claw marks down its back." I picked it up, along with some fabulous tools, through Al-Anon. This 12-step program was founded in the 1950's by the wife of Bill W., the founder of Alcoholics Anonymous. Bill's wife realized that *she* had issues from living with an alcoholic, and has helped many of us who have a friend or loved one or coworker who's an alcoholic. Given the fact that virtually all of us know someone with a drinking problem, I believe nearly all of us could benefit from Al-Anon.

For me, attending meetings and working the 12 steps ceased to be about the drug addict I was trying to control after the first few years. Now I use Al-Anon for great support, almost like free therapy, to learn how to move the mini-mountains that are truly mine and let the rest go. If letting go has been an issue for you, too, consider this helpful tool and know you can choose your own "Higher Power," rather than having to find a religious connection you may or may not feel.

Same day, 10 P.M. I'm stunned by the coincidence of what I wrote earlier—the first time I've put a date on something in this manuscript (and with good reason as I've been working on it nearly nine years). My friend and I had a blast after her return from a day on the slopes, drinking pomegranate martinis and consuming divine food at a favorite local restaurant. While in the Ladies' Room prior to my departure, I felt drawn to check my voice mail. There was an urgent message from Mom. I

knew it was not good news due to her fervent request that
I call her yet tonight. Hmmm....she never says that.
Rarely, I'll have to say now.

Her news was that my precious friend Debrah, a year
younger than I at 48, died tonight, leaving twin girls six
months old, and a husband of only two months. After several weeks of surgeries, serious infection, and finally heart
failure—in a fit, formerly-healthy woman—I believe the
true cause of her death was decades of conventional medical practice being short-sighted about antibiotics. Yes, I
know those drugs have saved the day in many instances;
but now, they are overused and often used inappropriately
as a knee-jerk preventative—just in case. One of the long-
term effects is the creation of superbugs, which are completely resistant to nearly all antibiotics................

I had to pause there for a deep breath. The real point
is that I need to let go of my illusion of control over the
immense ignorance and cloaking of Hippocrates' creed,
"First Do No Harm." To be accurate, from *Epidemics*, Bk. I,
Sect. XI, a translation reads:

> "Declare the past, diagnose the present, foretell
> the future; practice these acts. As to diseases,
> make a habit of two things—to help, or at least
> to do no harm."

Pharmaceutical drugs and surgery are—at rare times—
helpful and sometimes even necessary. But due to their
invasive nature, subsequent risks and side effects, I consider them to be an absolute last resort—after exploring

many other alternatives, with prayer as your guide, when choices need to be made.

Even with cancer, many people's greatest fear, you almost always have two to three weeks to gather information and other opinions before deciding on a protocol you believe in and are committed to. And if you happen to quit a stressful job you've hated for years while exploring those choices, you might just be halfway to healing. Don't let any health care practitioner, including me, unduly influence you or pressure you into following a path which doesn't feel right to you—or needs more prayer and reflection before a decision is made.

I'm not suggesting you float off through a field of daisies with nothing more than positive thoughts to help you heal your health imbalances. But for *my* body, I am starting to wait longer before I even take herbs—easily pulled from my office dispensary—in order to allow my body to follow its intuitive healing nature without interference. If I've been nurturing that nature well in the ways described in this book, my body will handle most issues well and quickly—especially if allowed to rest from other activities.

Even the crab has to let go of the shiny trinket he thought was a prize in order to get his daily food share. Celebrate this moment by reflecting on anything you have to be grateful for. If you can't come up with three things you're grateful for, go to an Al-Anon meeting.

Chapter Six

Special Issues
for Men

"The rule I use is, if it doesn't come out of the ground
looking the way it looks when you eat it, be careful.
There's no such thing as a PowerBar tree."

Dr. Mehmet Oz
Esquire Magazine, October 4, 2007

David was 46 when he first came to see me about chronic sinus congestion due to allergies. In terms of symptom relief, this is a pretty easy one to deal with using herbs like goldenrod, yerba santa and licorice root. Then we discovered some positive side effects for David from the licorice. He noticed having more energy and better sleep due to that plant's ability to support his stressed-out adrenals. Having less daily fatigue helped David get back to regular exercise which, in turn, helped ease his depression and provide even more energy for him.

However, he still had not been able to drop the extra 25 pounds he'd been carrying since starting his own business and working a lot of hours. Each time I spoke with him, I asked about his food diary which he hadn't found time for until he started feeling better. Once we reviewed his daily food choices, I had some great news for him regarding his weight: he wasn't eating enough! Like many people, David was enjoying a daily mocha latte on his way to work—his only breakfast—and lunch usually didn't happen due to his busyness. When he arrived home for dinner, he was starved and would grab whatever was fast and easy (junk food) to tide him over until his wife had dinner on the table.

Enjoying a sugar-laden caffeine drink for breakfast and nothing for lunch is only helpful for those who want to *gain* weight and don't care how they do it. When you go for long periods without eating, not only do you do a number on your blood sugar (which can contribute to diabetes), but you also give your body the message that starvation is near. Your body's goal then becomes hanging on to as much fuel (fat) as possible. This can contribute to depression and a host of other issues. After David started making a three-minute smoothie to drink on the way to work, taking a short break to eat a healthy lunch and snacking on things like celery sticks with peanut butter to tide him over at dinnertime, the weight dropped off in just a few months. He became a lot less cranky and more efficient at work, too.

Before I outline specific support on male issues, I want to acknowledge you for even reading this book, given my female perspective on health. Since I don't live in a man's body and consequently have not had to deal with the unique physical aspects of being a man, I offer the following ideas with humility and respect. That being said, several of my most significant herbal medicine teachers are men who have taught me a great deal about health in general, and men's health specifically.

You may not read the Special Issues for Women chapter, so if it makes you feel any better, I shop—and often think—like a guy. In fact, when my husband, Webb, and I recently gutted and updated a condo together in Steamboat Springs, Colorado using 95 percent recycled items from the Habitat for Humanity store, Craig's List and eBay, one of the maintenance guys made an interesting comment. After witnessing the two of us hauling appliances in and out of our second-floor unit, he said to Webb, "Boy, you sure do ask a lot of your wife." Webb's response was "Ya know…sometimes, she's more of a man than I am."

I feel like an honored guest in this chapter. Any wisdom you find in this chapter is thanks to many teachers,

Webb and my first two husbands among them. It's my belief that men and women in this day and age are making significant improvements in communicating with and understanding each other, creating improved health and happiness for all of us. I hope some of the simple tips in this chapter will help further that goal.

Statistically speaking, women live longer than men. I believe women's longevity has a lot to do with their paying attention to their health imbalances before something major happens. We're programmed from puberty to go to the doctor every year for an annual exam, whereas men often wait until they have a heart attack or are diagnosed with cancer—usually of the prostate—before they consider how their everyday choices might affect their health. Given that you are reading this, I think that bad habit is starting to change, "one guy at a time." And for all the ladies reading this chapter in order to convince your man to get his health act together, just remember, "the best sermon is a good example."

79. *Vitality Without Viagra—Erectile Dysfunction*

It is well documented that sex is on a man's mind most hours of the day, so let's just deal with this one right up front. According to *Rosemary Gladstar's Family Herbal*, 40 percent of sexually active men struggle with ED. Given that a large percentage of my male clients contact me about this very issue, that doesn't surprise me. But rather than just attributing it to aging (come on…in your 40s?), I think it's an accurate reflection of the toll that our stressful lifestyle takes on us. If you haven't read Chapter One on good, nourishing food, that's the place to start. However, if you're expecting only vegetarian recipes with a lot of hard-to-pronounce herbs and spices, you'll be happy to know that's not the case. Quality red meat is essential in most diets, but especially for men who need plenty of Vitamin B12 for energy and vitality.

Now for the shocking news: I want you to make an appointment with your physician at the same time you're making good-tasting dietary improvements to help correct this problem. Since lack of blood flow to the penis can sometimes parallel lack of blood flow to the heart, get that awesome muscle checked out soon—especially if you're considering buying Viagra or Cialis, which can exacerbate heart problems. If your doc gives you a hard time about the eggs and red meat I suggest, insist he or she check out *WestonAPrice.org* and don't budge on the recommended diet before they spend time on that website. We have all been sold a bill of goods by the food industry and "Big Pharm" regarding fat and the choles-terol craze. You'll find well-researched information on this debate at the Weston Price website.

Ten SuperFoods for Men

Food	*Benefit*
red meat*	protein and B12
yogurt and other fermented foods	aids digestion; supports immune function
dark-green leafy vegetables	great source of minerals, vitamins, fiber; protective against prostate cancer
wild (not farmed) fish	protein and essential fatty acids
lemon-flavored cod liver oil	primo food source of Vitamins A & D
pumpkin seeds	high in zinc; excellent for prostate
squash seeds	high in zinc; supports male glandular system and prostate
nettle tea	highly supportive of adrenal glands
eggs** (best raw or lightly cooked)	high in Vitamins B12 and D
hawthorn berries	super supportive of the heart

*only a SuperFood if grass-fed beef without hormones or antibiotics.
**only a SuperFood if the chickens can roam in the sun for Vitamin D and are given no hormones or antibiotics. Salmonella is extremely rare in these eggs.

The SuperFoods listed previously are great support for your overall health, but if I had titled this tip "Maintaining Vitality," would you have read it? A note on the hawthorn berries: they're not available as a crop so look for a solid extract in your local health food store or go to *herbalist-alchemist.com* for a reliable and high-quality source.

Achieving and/or maintaining an erection often has to do with stressed-out adrenal glands—or maybe just stress, in general. Since the adrenals of nearly all Westerners are severely depleted by age 40, drinking strong nettle tea (see #58 for instructions) is the perfect Super-Food to start with when you're having difficulty in the bedroom.

If you feel less attractive than when you and your partner first started doing the Wild Thing, you'll like the side effects of nettle tea: thicker and more lustrous hair, stronger nails without ridges (the ridges indicate lack of minerals), and skin that is blemish-free. Are you unsure about the taste of that highly-beneficial nettle tea? Add some fresh lemon or a bit of raw honey—heck, if it'll help you drink it, add some whiskey! Yes, I'm serious.

And just as a reminder, are you:

- ◆ Exercising vigorously (but not over-doing it) nearly every day?
- ◆ Eating plenty of fresh, raw veggies and high-quality protein at every meal?
- ◆ Taking one to two teaspoons daily of lemon-flavored cod liver oil?

◆ Eating something every 3½ hours to keep blood sugar levels even?

◆ Including ginger, cinnamon or garlic each day to enhance circulation?

◆ Limiting alcohol to one, sometimes two, beers or glasses of wine a day?

◆ Drinking one to two quarts of water daily in addition to nettle tea?

We're almost there. But before I reveal specific herbs for ED (erectile dysfunction) in guy form (a tincture that only requires a teaspoonful as opposed to a daily quart of nettle tea), we need to talk, or you need to read. Foreplay doesn't start five minutes before you want to have intercourse; it starts when you unload the dishwasher in the morning without being asked. And it continues when you pick up the kids from soccer, volunteer to handle dinner A to Z once a week, and give your woman a serious compliment about something you find gorgeous about her—hours before you want to "jump her bones." And, at the risk of freaking out all of you closet homophobes, these things also work if your partner is male.

Now, as Jack Nicholson would say…"Who's the lucky boy?" Still not quite happening, you say, after eating all those SuperFoods and drinking your nettle tea daily for a couple months? Even when you're practicing the prescribed foreplay hours before the hoped-for event? Okay, you've been good. Let's pull out the herbal big guns.

As always, it's best to work with a skilled practitioner who can provide a customized formula just for you. Ask

him or her about the following herbs to help when you
need a little something extra: Siberian ginseng, astragalus
root, ashwagandha, oats, dandelion, sarsaparilla and wild
yam. Licorice is also helpful—and increases your energy
level, too—but if you have high blood pressure, you simply must work with an experienced practitioner to make
sure it doesn't elevate your BP. And finally, I'll mention
saw palmetto which, as you are about to learn, is numero
uno in supporting a healthy prostate, in addition to sexual
function.

80. Ask for Directions—
Or Why Men Die Sooner

Okay, you won't really die sooner just because you don't
ask for directions, but the concept holds true. My belief
is that you testosterone-laden people usually don't ask for
directions because your hind-brain kicks in with the
thought that you are on your own and can rely on no one.
In a way, that's true; but when you fail to ask for help, it
places additional stress on you. Combine that with your
innate desire to always look cool (think Tony Manero in
Saturday Night Fever) and you might just find a long-term
recipe for a heart attack. Ironically, your female partner
will feel flattered if you ask for help occasionally, leading
to improved communication. And guess what *that* sometimes leads to?

81. *Your Pesky Prostate*

Most physicians will tell you that if you live long enough, you'll probably get prostate cancer. It's by far the most common type of cancer in men, but here's the good news: it might prolong your life. There's nothing like a cancer diagnosis to make you wake up and take better care of yourself with healthy nutrition and exercise. Those recommended, daily habits will also help prevent heart disease, which is the number one killer of both men and women. More good news is that prostate cancer almost always grows very slowly. I've had oncologists tell me that something else will likely kill you before prostate cancer advances enough to do so.

A chestnut-shaped organ no larger than a walnut, the prostate is part muscle and part gland, located below the bladder and next to the rectum. Makes you long for that next rectal exam, doesn't it? Well, get over it, guys; we women have docs going places with cold speculums on a regular basis from the time we're teenagers. But I digress.

If the prostate becomes inflamed or engorged, it squeezes the urethra which can lead to urinary incontinence or kidney infections. Prostatitis is inflammation of the prostate, often as a result of a low-grade urinary tract infection. If you receive a diagnosis of prostatitis that your physician believes originated in a urinary tract infection, consider herbal alternatives to an antibiotic. You'll find details in Chapter Five, #73, on bladder infections. Also check out the box below on Epsom salt therapy.

A more common issue is benign prostatic hyperplasia (BPH), when the prostate is enlarged; but it's not usually due to an infection. The symptoms of prostatitis and BPH are very similar:

◆ having to get up at night to urinate
◆ difficulty emptying the bladder completely
◆ painful urination
◆ reduced force when urinating
◆ unexplained chills and fever
◆ pain upon sitting
◆ blood in the urine (this is rare)

BPH symptoms are experienced by nearly 60 percent of North American males between the ages of 40 and 60. The causes are varied, but most are directly related to stress and diet. Eliminating or greatly reducing wheat and sugar is my best tip to reduce inflammation throughout your body. This is important since every major disease has inflammation as a component. Now, I know letting go of sugar and wheat isn't easy, so I'll give you a treat. Guess what helps the prostate and all your sexual organs to function more effectively? Two to four orgasms per week. Yup, that old adage is true: use it or lose it. And no, it does not have to include a partner, although that is my personal preference.

Prostate problems usually respond incredibly well to home treatment which includes dietary changes, herbal remedies and lifestyle changes. However, if your symptoms don't improve within a week, seek help from your holistic health care practitioner or physician. If your only symptom is blood in the urine, don't wait to make an appointment since that can be an indicator of bladder cancer. It's common for men to ignore symptoms until things get a lot worse. Be smart and listen to your body.

Now that you're listening, let's learn to use food as medicine. My preference is to focus mostly on what we *want* to eat for healing purposes, rather than a big list of forbidden foods. However, there are three things the prostate finds particularly irritating: alcohol, caffeine-rich foods and sugar. Do your best to eliminate them for a few weeks to make your prostate happy; then consider those items as an occasional treat. If you haven't read Chapter One on nutrition yet, start with the basics: lots of vegetables, quality protein—such as grass-fed beef or fish or beans—at each meal, plenty of fresh garlic taken with food, and soups with a bone-broth base, like chicken soup. Add medicinal herbs to your soups; for example, ginseng, astragalus root, and Shitake mushrooms all fortify your immune response. Finally, there are two beverages I'd like you to enjoy every day for prostate health: fresh lemon in water and unsweetened cranberry juice. However, you'll need to dilute the latter to make it palatable; four ounces of unsweetened cranberry juice to 28 or more ounces of water is what I suggest.

There are several specific foods that are excellent for reducing enlargement and inflammation of the prostate. They include:

◆ Pumpkin seeds (¼ to ½ cup daily; roast in butter if you like and add dried cranberries and raw sunflower seeds for a tasty alternative to chips)
◆ Cucumbers (two to three daily)

◆ Apples and onions, since both contain quercetin which helps limit cancer growth

◆ Stinging Nettles (freshly cooked or see #58 for a nettle tea recipe). You'll want to drink a quart daily until symptoms are gone, then one to two cups a day)

One reason I emphasize fresh nettles or nettle tea is for the many minerals you'll get in this nutrition-packed plant. One quart of nettle tea contains 2,000 milligrams of calcium plus generous amounts of bone-building magnesium, potassium, silicon, boron, and zinc. It is also an excellent source of Vitamins A, D, E and K. Vitamin K is especially important for a healthy prostate and can be found in dark, leafy greens and fermented foods and beverages. Sauerkraut, fermented chutneys or kombucha (a delicious drink) are a few examples of fermented foods that offer Vitamin K and a host of other benefits. Yes, beer is a fermented beverage with lots of B Vitamins, but alcohol needs to be enjoyed in moderation.

Mediterranean men consume the most cooked tomatoes worldwide, and have the lowest incidence of prostate cancer in the world; I suggest enjoying them several times a week—especially since tomatoes are known to help prevent heart disease, too. Using food as medicine costs a lot less than a handful of supplements, most of which are synthetic and expensive.

According to *Rosemary Gladstar's Family Herbal*, the two most important nutrients needed to prevent and help heal prostate cancer are Vitamins K and D. The greens and fermented items cover the Vitamin K; Vitamin D is easily handled with 15 minutes of sunshine a day without sunscreen or sunglasses (they prohibit Vitamin D from being absorbed through your eyes which is the best place for absorption). Wearing a hat will not prevent Vitamin D absorption.

What About Saw Palmetto?

Though saw palmetto alone may not be a "cure" for prostate cancer, it has been shown to be preventative and is certainly part of any adjunct therapy I recommend for those with prostate cancer who choose radiation or

Epsom Salts to the Rescue!

I'd like to give Thomas Cowan, M.D. credit for this simple suggestion. Given that the prostate is a muscular gland, you can treat acute prostatitis or an enlarged prostate the same way you treat other strained and inflamed muscles—with rest and Epsom salts. Soak in a warm or hot bath with one cup of Epsom salts for 20 minutes, twice a day for 10 days. The Epsom salts help cleanse the prostate by promoting secretion of its contents. The hard part is that ejaculation should be avoided for at least two weeks, but it will be worth it. Many patients experience immediate relief with this intensive bath therapy. See *westonaprice.org/men/ironmask* for more details.

chemotherapy. Thought of for centuries as the classic plant to reduce inflammation and irritation of the prostate, saw palmetto will also help increase your "reproductive qi" (pronounced "chee"), increasing fertility and minimizing problems with erectile dysfunction. You can use saw palmetto as a simple herb (by itself), but I prefer herbal formulas that you and your health care practitioner can customize for your needs.

If you choose chemotherapy or radioactive seeds as part of a cancer treatment protocol, you'll also want to include herbs like barberry root and leaf, Oregon grape root, Siberian ginseng or turmeric to enhance the efficacy of your modern medicine treatment. See David Winston's article, "Treatment of Bacterial MDR (Multiple Drug Resistance) with Botanical Therapies" in the Bibliography.

However, work with your health care practitioner to avoid potentially negative herb-drug interactions. To balance urinary flow, ask your practitioner about herbs like corn silk, nettle root or seeds, cleavers and uva ursi. Herbs to ease inflammation and congestion of the prostate include marshmallow root, echinacea and gravel root, in addition to the saw palmetto.

Many educated physicians now recommend herbal therapies as part of their treatment protocol. That's how I started working with a group of oncologists led by Mike Fangman, M.D., who is fabulous. He invited me to a meeting where I shared how we could integrate my work with theirs. I admired Dr. Fangman, and the other oncologists in his practice who were open-minded, for putting the best interest of their patients first; a great example of "integrative medicine." And I'm sure they didn't want the liability when their patients showed up with a grocery bag full of supplements with the question, "Is it okay if I take these herbs and supplements while on chemo, doc?"

Why do so many Americans think that modern medicine and herbal medicine are "alternatives" to one another? It's not either/or; it's not which is better, bigger, stronger, more successful (in terms of results) than "the alternative." Be wise; blend the best of both worlds. Consider modern medicine for diagnostics and emergency first aid; food, exercise and herbs for prevention; modern medicine again when you just have to have a Big Gun (like type I diabetes).

I'm sharing this information about preventing prostate cancer before a diagnosis discussion for a reason: get after these healthy habits *before* you have symptoms or receive a diagnosis. You have the power right now to take wise precautions for cancer prevention, which will also help prevent other diseases—like the number one killer, heart disease. If you have BPH symptoms already and are contemplating a medical appointment, consider the following details about testing as you gather information. Even rapidly growing cancers, which are rare in the prostate, can wait for two to three weeks while you collect information from various members of your health care team. And if you're advised to follow any invasive protocol immediately, I urge caution.

Before deciding on the best protocol, I invite you to…pray for guidance. You don't have to get religion, just stillness. Especially in this whipped-into-a-frenzy world of technology and instant decisions, it's best to center yourself first with your breath, and then ask for guidance from whatever you see as being smarter than humans. Maybe Nature? God (Good Orderly Direction)? If that type of language is as foreign to you as "medical speak," see Items #41, 42, 43 and 45 in Chapter Three.

Testing Options

◆ *PSA (Prostate-Specific Antigen)* There is much controversy about the value of prostate cancer screening, appropriate staging evaluation and optimal treatment for each stage of the disease. PSA tests have become a common diagnostic measure recommended to all men past 40, and, as a result, more early-stage cancers have been detected. However, this has not resulted in a lower mortality rate. (See Bibliography for two sources: Donald Yance's book, *Herbal Medicine, Healing and Cancer* and the article by Dr. David Williams, "True New Miracles for Men.")

A new development promises more accurate PSA testing through two types of PSA—free and protein-bound. A low ratio of free PSA to protein-bound PSA indicates the presence of prostate cancer with 95 percent accuracy; a high ratio indicates a benign condition. This may also minimize the confusion over elevated PSA levels due to other conditions such as acute hepatitis, low testosterone levels or an underlying liver disease.

◆ *TRUS (Transrectal Ultrasonography)* This new testing method uses a rectal probe to pass sound

waves from the probe to the prostate gland.
Since cancer cells differ from regular cells in the
way they absorb sound waves, the distinct
patterns of cancer cells indicate the presence of
prostate cancer. This type of testing is not
available everywhere, but is becoming
increasingly more popular since it is quite
accurate and far less invasive than biopsies.
You'll find more information on this at
www.cancerscan.com. TRUS is the first line
of diagnosis in other countries, but can be
difficult to find in the U.S.

◆ *Biopsies* This surgical option for diagnosis is
often recommended when the PSA is elevated or
a digital exam of the rectum by your physician
reveals an enlarged prostate. I'm not a big fan of
biopsies which can disturb the cancer, causing it
to grow more rapidly and/or spread to other
areas. These surgeries may also damage the
prostate, and definitely expose you to a possible
virus or bacteria which doesn't respond to
antibiotics. However, if you're an extreme
worrier and would be stressed without knowing
for sure, you may want to go this route.

Rosemary Gladstar's Family Herbal states, "the latest
findings suggest that men live the same length of time
with or without the surgery, but have much greater
discomfort with the surgery." Not to mention probable
erectile dysfunction. This does not mean surgery is
wrong for you if you find yourself with prostate

cancer—but it certainly gives credence to working with herbs and food as medicine for two to three months before making that decision.

Wow, that's a lot of prostate information; but given the statistics, this is the one issue I bring up with every

---

A Lesson in PSA Testing

from "True New Miracles for Men"
by Dr. David Williams

PSA is produced by all cells in the prostate gland, but malignant cells leak roughly ten times as much PSA into the bloodstream as do normal cells. Though many U.S. urologists believe that biopsies should be performed on a male of any age who has a PSA level of 4.0 ng/ml or higher, it's very common for the prostate to increase in size as men age, corresponding to increased PSA levels as you get older. The following PSA levels are the maximum that most men should have:

- 40-49 years of age, 2.5 ng/ml
- 50-59 years of age, 3.5 ng/ml
- 60-69 years of age, 5.0 ng/ml
- 70-79 years of age, 6.5 ng/ml

PSA levels should be used only as a guideline since only about 75 percent of men with prostate cancer have correspondingly elevated levels of PSA.

male client since prevention can make a big difference—and help you live a healthier life in all ways. If nothing else, include the foods listed above to reduce inflammation on a regular basis, exercise five times a week and start taking saw palmetto tincture once you reach age 45 or 50.

82. Sports and Their Everyday Injuries— Also Applicable for Women Weekend Warriors and Nice Nerds with Carpel Tunnel Syndrome

One thing I love about men is the teamwork they display at their best, often on a playing field. Athletics are more balanced now, but in the sixties and seventies when I was a kid, team sports were unusual for girls. Though the competitive nature of those with excess testosterone can become imbalanced, it also can keep you motivated to practice your skills. When my yoga students say, "I could never do that," while observing a pose, I remind them it took years of practice. For four years I spent a fair amount of time with my bum in the air and toes inching up toward my nose before actually being able to do a headstand. I often joke that my specialty, in terms of yoga students, are mid-life men who think they're too stiff to practice yoga. As soon as they see an improvement in their golf or basketball game after a few classes, they're hooked.

You may think this is a digression, but I'm right on track with my first tip for helping you to:

- ◆ improve your strength, flexibility and balance in any physical activity.
- ◆ recover from injuries, sports-related or otherwise, much faster.
- ◆ look 10-20 pounds thinner in three breaths (hint: posture).

◆ minimize or completely heal low-back pain which hits almost everyone by age 40.

◆ increase your awareness of everything, from how your body feels when you eat certain things, to the negative emotions you can release with greater ease.

If you haven't guessed yet, it's yoga. And please don't say to yourself, "Oh, no, I can't do yoga, I'm just not flexible." That's the point, handsome! You'll get more flexible no matter where you start, but choose the right teacher. Try various beginner classes until you find a teacher who honors your ability to say "no" to certain poses that don't feel right for you—and who celebrates your successes.

Sprains and Strains

Sprains occur when the ligaments around joints, such as wrists and ankles, over-stretch and sometimes even tear. If you're in the wilderness and have to wait for treatment, the best "first thing" to do is put the injured limb in water, preferably the cool, running water of a stream. According to Cascade Anderson Geller, a wise and respected herbalist in Portland, Oregon, water itself is very healing, and often the best place to start.

Though ice is overused in the West, it can be helpful in the first 24-48 hours. The best thing about it is it forces you to rest while you're icing. It also helps manage swelling and pain. However, swelling can actually be your friend with acute injuries since it increases circulation, providing more white blood cells to the injured area of your body. Start by applying ice (a frozen bag of peas or berries is my favorite) for 20 minutes, switch to a heating pad (preferably a rice bag heated in the microwave or a hot water bottle rather than an electric heating pad) for another 20 minutes. Shift back and forth between cold and heat, always ending with heat. You may also want to:

◆ apply a compress (crushed herbs) under the ice or heat to contain bruising. Choose from, or combine: distilled witch hazel, arnica, calendula, yarrow, or St. John's wort (use one to two teaspoons of tincture in a little water if fresh plant is unavailable). Or you can place the inner side of a banana peel directly on the bruise.

◆ take the same remedy internally that you use on the compress; three droppersful (90 drops) in a little water immediately, then one dropperful (30 drops) every two to four hours.

◆ support the sprained joint with a bandage, "ace" or otherwise.

◆ rest! Let your body use your energy for healing, rather than busyness; this is a great time to catch up on reading.

◆ consult your physician if the pain has not improved considerably after 24 hours, since the underlying bone may be broken. Lovely.

83. The Cholesterol Crock

Americans have been brainwashed by the food industry about fats being bad for us, and further programmed to believe that having total cholesterol (TC) under 200 is necessary for heart health. But consider this: people with "high" total cholesterol live the longest! Incredible, but true. Having TC that is too low has many negative implications, especially regarding longevity and fertility. To read scientific papers demonstrating that the key to a happy heart and long life is not necessarily having low total cholesterol, check out the following website: *WestonAPrice.org/moderndiseases/benefits_cholest.html.*

Even among those who believe high cholesterol automatically leads to heart disease, most agree that the *ratio* of TC (total cholesterol) to HDL(high density lipids) cholesterol, and your triglycerides number are far better measures. An average TC to HDL ratio is 4.5, but the best would be 2 or 3 or at least under 4. For triglycerides, less than 150 mg/dl is considered normal; under 100 is ideal.

The latter finding was confirmed by Dr. Rauchhaus, in cooperation with other researchers at several German and British university hospitals. They found that the risk of dying for patients with chronic heart failure was strongly and inversely associated with total cholesterol, LDL cholesterol and triglycerides; those with high lipid values lived much longer than those with low values. Learn more at *ncbi.nlm.nih.gov/pubmed/14662255.*

Other researchers have made similar observations. The largest study was performed by Professor Gregg C. Fonorow and his team at the UCLA Department of Medicine and Cardiomyopathy Center in Los Angeles. The study, led by Dr. Tamara Horwich, included more than a thousand patients with severe heart failure. After five years, 62 percent of the patients with cholesterol below 129 mg/l had died, but only half as many of the patients with cholesterol above 223 mg/l were no longer with us. For more information on this, check out *WestonAPrice.org/moderndiseases/ benefits_cholest.html*

A better indicator of potential heart disease than cholesterol is the C-Reactive Protein test which measures inflammation in your body—a common link with all major diseases. To more accurately determine your risk, ask your physician about getting this test. You'll soon read more about it in the news.

High Cholesterol Protects Against Infection

Many studies have found that low cholesterol can be worse than high cholesterol. For instance, in 19 large studies of more than 68,000 deaths, reviewed by Professor David R. Jacobs and his co-workers from the Division of Epidemiology at the University of Minnesota, low cholesterol predicted an increased risk of dying from gastrointestinal and respiratory diseases.

A number of pathogens have been associated with the development of CHD (Coronary Heart Disease) or have been found in the atherosclerotic lesions at autopsy, including both viruses and bacteria. These pathogens have been around as long as man has lived on the earth. The culprit, therefore, is not the microbes but a compromised immune system which can no longer deal with them appropriately. A healthy immune system depends on an array of nutrients, including Vitamin A, Vitamin C and various minerals.

One of the most tragic aspects of the cholesterol campaign is that it has caused Americans and Europeans to abandon fats that provide protection against infection. Not only do animal fats carry Vitamin A, they also contain palmitoleic acid, a 16-carbon monounsaturated fatty acid that has strong antimicrobial properties. Butterfat and coconut oil contain fatty acids that have similar properties. They protect against viruses and pathogenic bacteria, plus enhance the immune system. Areas of the world where coconut milk and oil is consumed have low levels of heart disease.

84. Creating and Maintaining a Happy, Healthy Heart

The great thing about heart disease is it's easy to reverse—with the right support. Though you may know that eating five servings a day of fresh vegetables and fruit can help prevent and reduce CHD and that exercise is critical, you may not consider one of the greatest contributors of heart disease—ignoring emotions. While training at The Chopra Center with Deepak Chopra, M.D. and Simon Mills, M.D., I heard Dr. Chopra say something so basic, yet so memorable: "The heart is so much more than just a big muscle that needs the right nourishment and exercise. It must be nourished from within."

The heart is an organ of fire, fed by love, touch, feeling and sensory experiences that many men lack. The workplace certainly doesn't support the "touchy-feely" stuff and often, home doesn't provide intimate heart energy either. Having male friends is important, though unfortunately, unless there's a true crisis, guys seem to connect through sports or a beer after work where the most intimate part of the discussion focuses on work. If you're not rolling your eyes and would like to explore this idea further, check out the works of Sam Keene and Robert Bly whose insights into the heart of a man are worthy of exploration. If you are rolling your eyes, never fear, we're shifting gears.

Food as Medicine for a Healthy Heart

You may have heard about some of the food tips which follow, but I want to start with one that might rock your world. Quality fat (yes, even some saturated fat) is good for you in a myriad of ways, including keeping your heart healthy. Stay with me here 'cause you're going to love this. The amount of fat in the typical American's diet has held fairly steady at 35 to 40 percent of calories for the last 90 years, while the rate of heart disease has been rising. The Masai tribe in Africa consumes 60 percent of their calories from fat and are *free* of heart disease. The traditional diet of the Eskimos and North American Indians was 80 percent fat, and there is no indication that they suffered from heart disease. Whereas, more currently in the U.S.:

◆ Between 1910 and 1970, the proportion of traditional animal fat in our diet declined from 83 percent to 62 percent.
◆ Butter consumption went from 18 pounds per person per year to four in that same period.
◆ Dietary cholesterol intake has increased only one percent during the past 80 years.
◆ During that same period of time, the percentage of dietary vegetable oils in the form of margarine, shortening and refined oils increased about 400 percent while the consumption of sugar and processed foods increased about 60 percent.

What these consumption patterns indicate is that the type or quality of fat matters. Ninety years ago, Americans consumed mostly animal fats—lard, butter and tallow from pasture-fed animals. These fats were stable and provided many important nutrients.

Today, most of the fats in the American diet are liquid vegetable oils or oils that have been hardened through the process of hydrogenation. A large fraction of calories from polyunsaturated vegetable oils are new to the human diet and we are the guinea pigs. These oils lack Vitamins A and D found in animal fats; cod liver oil, however, is well-known for a beautiful combination of these important Vitamins (and taste need not be an issue with a bit of lemon added).

Those who are trying to avoid eating lots of fat often replace fat calories with calories from refined flour and sugar. Several researchers have published studies linking consumption of refined carbohydrates, particularly sugar, with increased heart disease, including Yudkin in the 1950s and Lopez in the 1960s. Yudkin found that use of sugar was associated with increased adhesiveness of the blood platelets, increased blood insulin levels and increased blood corticosteroid levels. **See the website at** *healthlibrary.com/reading/health/3chap2.*

To be proactive, try the following for heart health and enjoy many positive side effects including more energy, less stress, fewer headaches and greater flexibility.

◆ Greatly reduce or eliminate processed sugar and refined white flours. This will significantly reduce inflammation in your entire body and make watching your weight infinitely easier. You'll likely get fewer winter colds, too. Not sure what a "whole" grain is? If any grain on a label does not have the word "whole" in front of it, it's processed. If you get confused, just eliminate wheat.

◆ Eat a wide variety of fruits and vegetables (think color) any way you like them. They contain various beta carotenes, the same ingredient (plus resveratrol) which makes red wine a healthy addition to your diet—in moderation. That means one or two glasses a day.

◆ Include plenty of tomatoes and tomato sauce in your diet; there's a reason why those guys in the Mediterranean have much lower incidence of heart disease.

For more information on quality fats, see #7, and also, check out the following web site: *WestonAPrice.org/moderndiseases/hd*.

Move Your Body

An article appeared in JAMA (Journal of the American Medical Association) some time ago stating that exercise is the number one predictor of heart disease—more important than whether or not you smoke. Wow. Make it a goal to move your body daily and be happy with at least 30 minutes four to five times a week with a variety of activities. If that still sounds overwhelming, start with just five minutes of daily walking, dancing or skipping. Okay, maybe stick to walking as you may not dance and some people still think real men don't skip.

Heart-Supportive Herbs

Nettle tea (#58) is a perfect example of consuming food as medicine. Although it's more specific to the adrenal glands than the heart, I like to start here for heart support since stressed-out adrenals contribute to many health imbalances. You guys carry a lot of responsibility on your shoulders and usually without complaining. Though this is one of the traits I value in men, it can contribute to heart disease when you forget that most of life's frustrations are "Small Stuff."

Start by supporting your adrenal glands, which are the number one area of stress impact, by drinking a daily quart of nettle tea—instead of one of the two to three quarts of water you're hopefully drinking each day. After a month or two of this maximum adrenal support, one to two cups a day will suffice for maintenance. And if you thought I was kidding about adding whiskey to nettle tea to get you to drink it, I'm not. Susun Weed, one of my valued teachers, is the one who said that if a bit of added whiskey is what it takes for you to drink it, the tremendous benefits are worth it.

In addition, consider adding one or more of the following herbs in easy-to-take tincture form: hawthorn berries, motherwort, chickweed, oat, wild cherry bark or yarrow. These herbs all support the heart, but hawthorn is the classic and has virtually no side effects. You can also consume hawthorn berries in a solid extract from *herbalist-alchemist.com* to enjoy as food. However, since hawthorn can actually increase the effectiveness of beta blockers and other heart medications, work with your doctor to reduce your dose of those pharmaceuticals. Kerry Bone, author of *The Essential Guide to Herbal Safety*, also suggests taking hawthorn two hours before or after the medication thiamine.

Motherwort is another favorite of mine for heart support, especially when an individual also struggles with eczema or chronic bronchitis, since it helps heal those health issues, too. Although typically thought of as a "woman's herb," motherwort is a specific remedy for those with cardiac deficiency or angina. It's also great on an energetic level when you need to find the strength of a mother bear protecting her cubs in order to say "no" and set limits. The only possible contraindication is during pregnancy, so not to worry if you're male.

85. *Blood Pressure Blues*

Though blood pressure is closely tied to heart concerns, we'll give this issue space of its own. The first recorded instance of the measurement of blood pressure was in 1733 (on a horse), but it was not until 1847 that human blood pressure was recorded. Modern medicine's use of this technique required the further invention of the stethoscope and the blood pressure cuff, so it wasn't until 1903 to 1910 that it became a common measurement at Massachusetts General Hospital, where systematic records of blood pressure were first kept in the U.S.

One of the reasons I like, and rely on, blood pressure measurement to determine possible heart concerns is because it's been used for a relatively long period of time. I don't want to be anyone's guinea pig, which is why I prefer herbs with centuries of empirical evidence to pharmaceuticals that have a few years of testing—at best—before receiving FDA approval.

Blood pressure measurement is completely non-invasive and has a high rate of accuracy, but have you noticed what Big Pharm is up to? After decades of 120/80 being the gold standard, they now tell us it should really be 115/75, which would result in millions more customers for their blood pressure-reducing drugs. Coincidence? I don't think so. And if you're like many of us forgetful folks, the upper number, which is larger, is called diastolic and the number underneath (which should be smaller) is called systolic. It's actually the systolic reading that we are most concerned with when it's elevated.

All the same guidelines for keeping your heart happy apply to maintaining a healthy blood pressure reading: wholesome food, regular exercise and heart-healthy herbs. But there is one herb which is the ultimate for supporting normal blood pressure and is nearly free since it's best taken in raw food form: garlic.

Garlic, which also helps your immune system fight off "bad" bacteria, viruses and fungi, is my number one favorite for helping to balance blood pressure and is a great demonstration of the difference between herbs and pharmaceutical drugs. Given that my blood pressure is typically 115 over 70 or so, if I took Diovan, a common medication prescribed to lower BP, it would force my body to lower my BP, possibly to a dangerously-low level. But if I started taking fresh garlic instead, my BP would remain unchanged since herbs support the body in finding its own balance rather than forcing it to make a change.

In addition to the digestive caution in the box on the next page, you must proceed with caution and professional guidance if you're on a synthetic blood thinner (like Coumadin). First contact your health care practitioner about using garlic to gradually wean off of the blood thinner. Gradually replacing a blood thinner with garlic not only helps keep your blood the right viscosity—without potentially harmful side effects—but as a natural antibiotic, antiviral, and antifungal remedy, it has a positive side effect: fewer colds and flu. I commonly work with physicians on this transition, which is not a big deal since regular blood work must be done, anyway, for someone on a synthetic blood thinner. If your doctor is not open to that discussion, it may be time to interview a new one.

Susan's Simple Tip

A garlic bud is made up of 10 or more garlic cloves. Mince a clove or two each morning, swallowing it off the end of a spoon with some water. A drop of honey can be added if the taste is an issue. But don't waste your money on garlic capsules since most have the odor removed which is the most medicinal part. **Caution:** if you have digestive problems, start very small with your daily garlic (perhaps one-tenth of a clove) and take it with food as you gradually increase the dose over several weeks. It will usually heal your digestive issues, too!

86. Birth Control—
Or How to Avoid Child Support

Part of the reason Western women get cranky around their monthly "Moon" is it gets really old to be in charge of birth control responsibilities, requesting STD test results from a new partner, pregnancy, childbirth, nursing and then the "adolescence in reverse" known as menopause. Not to mention scrubbing toilets. Now, I ask you—wouldn't that give *you* PMS?

Seriously, though, did you know that Native American women have historically had almost zero incidences of Premenstrual Syndrome (PMS)? They're the ones who used a Moon Lodge where they all cycled together monthly, joining each other in the same tipi to sing, laugh, pray, ask each other for advice and basically chill for five days. During that time, their husbands/fathers/boyfriends/sons took over on all the home-tending duties. Hmmmm......what a concept. If you want to score big-time with your lady, offer to do every household duty possible during at least one day each month—and let her choose the day.

There are some herbs that the old Materia Medicas say reduce or eliminate active sperm count, but I would not put your faith in that route. Tip #75 reviews a woman's family planning choices, so educate yourself before having a discussion with your partner. To be precise, condoms are 86 to 97 percent effective at preventing pregnancy, depending on how they are used, so be wise. Use them in conjunction with another barrier method—or two.

87. STD's/STI's—What You Don't Know Could Kill Your Partner

Do you like how this chapter starts and ends with sex? That's the guy part of me. It also increases the likelihood of you reading, or at least skimming, the whole chapter.

The first step is communication, every man's favorite thing—especially when dealing with the details of sexual pleasure. If you want to score lots of points with a potential new partner, *you* be the one to initiate that little chat before having sex. This means talking with her (assuming you're straight) about preventing sexually transmitted infections (STI's) and pregnancy with choices that respect both of you.

Not being a fan of synthetically altering a woman's hormones for decades, I consider birth control pills to be a short-term solution of five to seven years—ten tops. I know it's simple and effective—plus a total no-brainer for you guys—but synthetic hormones are known to contribute to breast cancer and other areas of concern for women, so get over it. If I'm going to help you with your sex life, you need to do your part by being responsible and awake.

The new term, sexually transmitted infection (STI), seems more accurate to me than sexually transmitted disease (STD) since most of these infections are fairly easy to get rid of—I emphasize *most* of them. But something like AIDS can kill you and belongs in that "disease" category. This needs to be the second topic of discussion with a new partner before actually doing The Wild Thing. Both of you should be prepared to exchange lab results to "prove" you're clean; if you haven't been that much of a Boy Scout, contact Planned Parenthood or your local county health office for information on testing.

In tip #73, I get into some details regarding HPV (Human Papillomavirus) and how some strains of this virus can lead to cervical cancer. This is why it is so critical for you guys to get tested. Since you can often have HPV, and other STI's, with zero symptoms, presenting your new partner with a recent negative lab report is an important pre-sex ritual. The HPV virus is tougher to get rid of than chlamydia, the most common STI these days. If you want to do it with herbs and lifestyle changes, that will require a trip to your herbalist or naturopath since it's too dicey of a topic for me to address here. That being said, there are many anti-infective herbs to assist with this issue.

88. Yeast Infections—Yes, Handsome, This Could Be Your Issue, Too

Huh? Why address yeast infections under men's health? Few women or men realize that, even though not technically an STI, partners can easily pass yeast back and forth to each other. If your wife or girlfriend is having repeated problems with this uncomfortable issue, you're likely to know it since sex is off limits and no fun for a woman with a yeast infection. Chapter Five, #69, gets into the specifics necessary for the female, but you guys can help a lot with two things:

◆ First, cut back on sugar (good for you, anyway) so that your seminal fluid won't contribute to the pH imbalance which can keep this infection going. The pH scale corresponds to the concentration of hydronium ions (H+) in a solution; too much sugar in the diet can increase its concentration.

◆ Second, follow these directions for prevention: When your partner repeatedly gets yeast infections, it's likely that even though you can't pick up the infection from her, you are passing it back to her as soon as she finishes her protocol to get over it. To prevent this, keep a spray bottle in the shower with the following solution in it: distilled water (or tap water if that's all that's available) with one tablespoon of **white distilled**

vinegar. After each shower, spray the diluted vinegar directly onto your genitals before you dry off. Keep this up for two to three weeks or until your partner no longer has this type of infection—and reap the rewards for being such a thoughtful and educated guy!

Chapter Seven

Time-Savers

"Time you enjoy wasting is not wasted."

—John Lennon

My awesome book shepard, Dr. Judith Briles, is convinced that it's money that keeps many of us from taking better care of ourselves, but I think it's a perceived lack of time. As a recovering workaholic who had a very warped relationship with time for the first 40+ years of life, I've often read books about how to get more done in less time. Then after perfecting the art of multitasking, I started studying yoga and meditation which suggests doing only one thing at a time. What's a good girl who prizes efficiency to do?

The big reality check arrived when my husband, Webb, asked me once what it is that I'm thinking about throughout the day as I perform both work and home tasks galore. "What I need to do next or what I should be doing instead," was my response. When I asked him the same question, he said "I think about what I'm doing." Yikes. I hate it sometimes when I hear the truth about my twisted approach to life. But it's actually been very helpful for me in my search to live in the present and enjoy life more—both of which are happening much more frequently, I'm happy to report.

Though I now see time differently after reading the amazing book on life, *A New Earth*, by Eckhart Tolle, I also recognize how easy it is to use a lot of hours on various activities just because *Vogue* magazine or our mothers told us to. If you haven't yet found the time to get some exercise daily or eat whole foods, this chapter is for you! Even if you only do half of what I suggest in the following tips, you'll have an extra eight to ten hours every week for self-care—which includes taking a nap or simply resting.

89. *Clean Less, Live More*

Many of us in the West, especially women, have a hyper-vigilant idea of what clean means. Think of how much time you would save if you lived by the philosophy "Clean enough to be healthy; Dirty enough to be happy." I've seen moms, and to a lesser degree, dads, get so compulsive about cleaning that it occupies the majority of their conversations with their children and spouses. Let's face it; no one wants to spend time with a nag. So rather than always reminding others to do more, or increasing your own stress level as you do it all, consider these tips:

- ◆ Do less laundry. Encourage your family to lessen the laundry load by wearing clothes again if they pass the sniff test. That's right; just take a sniff under the arms. If you're not offended, no one else will be. If you can't convince your kids to do this, or to use the same towel and washcloth for a week, just have them fold the clothes a time or two and this issue is a done deal.

  My mother always thought sheets should be washed once a week. One of my mothers-in-law also believed they should be *ironed*. This must have been a 50's thing when very few women worked outside the home or had their own businesses. If you take a shower or bath every night, the sheets can easily go two weeks and, I can testify, they do not walk on their own after three. You're clean when you get in there, and unless you have frequent and really creative sex, they just don't get dirty that quickly. And ironing the sheets? Please—only if the Queen of England is coming for a visit. But, I think she'd be happier in a local hotel.

◆ Let the dust go and re-evaluate how clean the floors really need to be. Both my hubby and I enjoy having a clean home, but since I find nearly anything else more exciting than housecleaning, and my husband doesn't like to have an outsider do the cleaning, we've learned to live with a dirtier house. When it bugs us, we clean, and only the parts that are bugging us. I found that by letting things go a bit longer, he somehow noticed when the toilet started forming a pink ring and would do it himself— hmmm...... This also provides a really good reason to entertain occasionally to stay connected with our friends. It's not that I'm cleaning *for* my friends, just using their visit as an excuse.

◆ If you're not convinced you can live in a dirtier house (and believe me, some of you shouldn't), invest in a copy of *Speed Cleaning* by Jeff Campbell. He gives great advice on how to do your housecleaning in less than half the time.

◆ Remove your shoes at the front door and have an attractive sign in the entry that invites your guests to do the same—especially if they're under four feet tall. This simple practice has many benefits: less dusting and vacuuming due to a huge reduction in dust and other bits; less noise around the house; and carpets that wear longer and need cleaning less often. But the greatest benefit is how this Asian practice helps you feel like you've entered your sanctuary when you arrive back home. You can even take a deep breath and literally leave your workday troubles at the door. I have a basket in the entry with slippers in it for clients and friends so they feel like they've been welcomed into our sanctuary rather than scolded for tracking in dirt.

90. *Streamline Your Face and Fashion*

Cut down on make-up—way down to simple base or powder with some lipstick. Over the past several years, I've let go of mascara and eye shadow except for a few special occasions. My husband actually likes it better and it shaves many minutes off my daily maintenance time. Next, find a cute and simple haircut that works well for your face and takes minimal time to style. If you don't trust your hairdresser to recommend something, find a new one by asking those you see with an attractive, low-maintenance cut, where they go. My stylist tells me that short hair can be easy and long hair can be easy, but those in-between styles can be time-consuming and frustrating.

Every woman and man has at least one simple and timeless style which will both look good and be ready to go in minutes. When I work out at the health club, I often notice women who are blow-drying their hair when I go in to take a steam and shower, and they are still blow-drying their hair when I walk out of the locker room completely dressed. What a drag! Having simpler hair will also serve you well when you want to travel, especially to a foreign country like Nepal, where they often don't even have electricity.

Be selective on shoes and accessories—yes, black really does go with everything. Brown is now the new black, but in general, if something doesn't go with black, red, or white I don't buy it—most of the time. Clearly this depends on your coloring, but if you have basic black worsted wool slacks, you can choose nearly any color blouse which is flattering to your face and coloring. If it's trendy, wait to buy it until part-way through the season when it's seriously discounted.

A fun blouse or scarf in this year's color is perfect with those timeless black slacks, and makes you feel up-to-date without having to change your wardrobe every year. I especially like to center my wardrobe around black when I'm traveling; it doesn't show soil and looks great with almost everything else in my wardrobe. And from a health perspective, high heels are out! A new study shows that the chunky heels are just as tough on your knees as the stilettos. Save one or two pair for very special occasions and find comfortable shoes for everything else.

Have you ever noticed how Oprah seems to wear those gorgeous diamond earrings almost daily, and they look perfect with everything? I'm not quite there yet—I'm still hooked on my various silver chains and pendants, but if you really want to save time and simplify, get a quality pair of silver or gold earrings, or some cubic zirconias (few can really tell the difference), and wear them every day. If you need another incentive, the "less is more" philosophy of jewelry is chic right now. Maybe our culture is finally coming to its senses. Yeah, right.

91. *Grocery Shopping in Half the Time*

When I was studying French at a language school in Vichy, France, I became enamored with their habit of stopping by the local market on the way home from work each day to purchase fresh food for the ensuing 24 hours. Living with a host family there (who spoke no English) in 2004 taught me the value of this simple practice— among other things. But in the U.S., I experience a faster pace with each new technological advance. Dealing with traffic and parking is stressful and time-consuming on its own; then the trip around the store, often at the busiest after-work time, is enough to make you want to eat fast food and blow off your workout.

Instead, consider borrowing a great idea from Elaine St. James' *Simplify Your Life* series. With a small, one-time investment of an hour or so, you can easily save hours each week. Start by typing a list of all the items you might possibly purchase. Then arrange them in the order they appear in the aisles of your favorite grocery store. If, like me, you shop at two different markets since the health food store doesn't carry everything, make two different lists. Save them on your computer and always keep a fresh printed list (or two) in one of your kitchen cabinets. It can easily be updated as your eating patterns change— and I fervently hope they will after reading this book.

As you use up something or realize you're getting low, check it off on your list. Your meal planning will be even easier if you're also using the Pantry Principle outlined in #10. Most of what you'll be checking off on your list will be fresh produce since you'll have the basics on hand. If you're on a budget—and who isn't?—take a look at the weekly flyer your market(s) distributes so you can stock up on basic pantry and freezer items when they're on sale.

The entire process, from making the list to doing the shopping to putting the groceries away, takes 60 to 90 minutes weekly for a family of four. You'll also save time by avoiding a last-minute trip to the store for forgotten items. Not only will you save hours each week which can be devoted to quiet time, exercise and making nettle tea, you'll save plenty of "buckage" to go toward your next vacation. As a bonus, if you are the main shopper and have to be out of town or just don't want to be responsible for marketing that week, you can hand the list over to your honey or old-enough-to-drive teenager.

92. Minimize All Shopping

I know some people just love to shop as a recreational activity—and have little spare time and hefty credit card balances as a result. For many, shopping is nothing more than another bad habit. Reminding myself that everything I buy today will someday end up in the landfill, helps me pause before buying. And I must admit, shopping is an area where I am more like a guy: I want to know what I want, have the money to buy it, go to the store and buy it, and come home to drink a beer on the patio.

Better yet is shopping online, though I do my best to support local businesses. I know many women think I'm cuckoo, but shopping is just not my gig—except at consignment stores, where I delight in finding designer clothes at a fraction of the retail price tag, which is sometimes still attached.

If you really need to shop for a particular item, take a friend along who's good at helping you police your purchases enough for you to buy only the intended item. Paying by cash or check reminds you of the true cost of things better than using a credit card (though many establishments don't even take checks anymore). You may have to work on breaking your addiction to reading every advertisement in the newspaper to reduce your shopping craving—and save more time. For an even greater time-saver, go on a news fast; most of it's negative anyway.

Create a list of other activities you can do when the shopping craving hits: have tea with a friend, take a walk, go to the library. Though you may feel deprived at first, you'll discover a freedom you've never known when you no longer feel that craving to buy. As an extra bonus, jot down the approximate amount you might have spent on each shopping excursion you resist for a year. I'll bet it's plenty for a vacation on the beach with your entire family.

93. *Turn Off the TV*

Studies indicate that most Americans have the television on for seven to eight hours each day—even though we all say we don't have time to exercise or cook. Not only does this consume time that is better spent elsewhere, it also affects your bank account (by buying more advertised stuff) and sleep (especially if you're in front of the TV the last hour before bed).

The first step is to keep a TV log of the programs you're watching, to get a reality check on the quantity and quality of your viewing. Then consider whether the sitcoms and repeated exposure to violence does anything to enhance your life. If you lead the way in determining which shows you can live without, and reward your children with time spent on their favorite games, you'll all win.

There are some programs that have merit, but before my husband and I were able to record them, I watched episodes of a favorite program that weren't all that great, just because it was 4:00 PM and I could pay bills at the same time. Now that our need for a new TV forced us get cable after 18 years without it, I spend even less time in front of the "boob tube." With DVR or TIVO, it's easy to scroll through to the episode of most interest, and eliminate others. I find this a more relaxing way to fold the laundry or go through stacks of mail.

If you suspect you might be addicted to TV, pick up a copy of *Unplugging the Plug-in Drug* by Marie Winn to learn about the true cost of all those hours in front of the box. It also offers simple ways to help you and your children reduce your watching hours or even break free completely. Those I know who have kicked the habit say it's one of the best things they've ever done.

While you're at it, you may want to cancel most or all of your magazine subscriptions, too, unless they truly enhance your life or educate you. We don't even have a newspaper subscription anymore. Instead, I took the advice of Timothy Ferris in *Four Hour Work Week*. I scan the headlines when I go past a newspaper dispenser, and then say to whomever I have a meeting with that day, "Hey, I haven't read the paper today; is there anything critical happening out there?"

94. Create Happier Holidays

If you like to read as much as I do, the place to start—for laughter as well as permission—is with *Skipping Christmas* by John Grisham. But you don't have to skip the holidays completely to save time and get back your sanity during a stressful time of year. The place to start is with decorations.

Before purchasing anything, drag out those Christmas boxes (which naturally are marked as such to minimize time spent in finding them) and use two empty ones to cull out what is ready for Goodwill and what you want to save for your children when they become young adults. Just because Aunt Sally gave you those porcelain angels a hundred years ago doesn't mean you still like them or have to keep them. Anything that didn't make it out of the Christmas box last year gets put into one of the other two boxes.

Select only the trim that you still like, that requires little or no dusting and is easy to put up and take back down. Minimize the number of rooms you add festive decorations to so you don't keep finding bits and pieces to go down to the basement in February. I love outdoor lights so I use some that are energy-efficient on our bushes. But I no longer wrap the tree trunk and branches with all those little lights that take forever to wind around the branches—only to have the whole thing fuzz out into darkness after the first two nights when a neighbor kid clips the cord for fun. I like to have a garland lining the edges of our front door. The one I use has been quick and easy to put up since I twined the lights around the fake greens several years ago and then left them together when I removed them in early January.

Now for the tough stuff: cards and gifts. I do enjoy sending and receiving holiday cards and letters, but find myself so swamped during the holidays that it becomes a chore rather than a pleasure. Instead, consider sending an annual update of family happenings as a Valentine's greeting after the holiday pressure is off; or maybe just prior to Thanksgiving as a way of giving thanks for the friends and family in your life.

A letter printed out on attractive and seasonally-appropriate paper is the least time-consuming and most personal way to connect, with brief notes added in the margin. I send them mostly to out-of-town friends, and it's a lot more fun when I'm not stressing about how to work this project into an already-groaning schedule.

Gift-giving can be simplified with a two-step process. For all gifts, I have a "gift closet" where I place things I find throughout the year that seem just right for a particular person's birthday or Christmas present. I also use it to store little hostess, housewarming and baby gifts that I find on sale. It's easy to find things 75 percent off or more directly after a holiday season; stock up on many of the same items when the cost is minimal. Rather than buying and storing expensive holiday wrapping papers, use leftover brown grocery bags turned inside out and cut into "sheets." Rubber stamps with various colored ink pads allow you to personalize packages. A bit of ribbon and you're set.

Holiday giving has become even simpler since I learned about organizations like Heifer International. They give you the chance to donate a few ducks, baby chicks, a lamb, goat, or cow to a family in need. The recipients in developing countries often become self-supporting by selling eggs, goat's milk and the like to others in their community. You can make a tax-deductible donation in honor of your loved ones and either print a card online indicating what you're giving in their name, or Heifer International will send you a more attractive version via snail mail. No driving, shopping, fighting crowds, gift-wrapping or waiting in line at the post office. Even my mom does this, to some degree, now—and she is the Queen of gift-giving and beautiful wrappings.

95. Get Up an Hour Earlier

I can hear you screeching, but the best hour of the day is the hour just before the time you currently get up. Most of us arise just in time to shower and dress, grab a quick bite to eat and take a look at the morning paper. If you have children to direct, that time is built-in, too. Stay with me here; I promise you won't end up sleep deprived if you follow some guidelines.

Imagine how scrumptious it would be if you had a whole extra hour in the morning to do what you really *want* to do, like taking a walk or having a little quiet time to gaze out at the bird feeder and just breathe, or read a great book, or write a thank-you note while listening to gentle music. Giving yourself this gift of time, especially if you use it for something other than work or email, is very effective for reducing your stress level. Your greater sense of peace helps you feel more sane, and you probably *will* be more sane—and more productive.

Not convinced yet? Consider how productive you are in the first few hours of a typical morning than you are in the last hour or two of your evening before you drop into bed. Now give yourself the gift of going to bed an hour earlier, especially if you're already feeling sleep-deprived. Most of us are unproductive and inefficient at the end of the day, and if you're like many who wake in the middle of the night and can't go back to sleep, you'll get an extra hour of deep sleep before that frustrating 2:00 A.M. wake-up time. Of course, you probably won't be waking without being able to go back to sleep after you start drinking a quart a day of nettle tea (#58). One more sleep treat: go to bed by 9:00 P.M. one night a week. I'm breathing more deeply just thinking about it.

If you still feel like there is never enough time in the day, pick up a copy of *Four Hour Work Week* by Timothy Ferris. His suggestion of checking email and voice mail only twice a day, at 10 A.M. and 4 P.M., has freed me up greatly to focus more on my own priorities, rather than other people's urgencies which are often due to lack of planning. Another idea he has to free up oodles of time is a 21st century version of delegating—via email. For a nominal hourly fee, you can secure virtual assistants through *Elance.com* to help with everything from planning and booking your next vacation or business trip, to creating a marketing brochure.

Parting Thoughts

It's a rough world out there, so I've done my best to keep these suggestions for your health gentle and manageable; but now it's time to kick butt—or bum, as I usually say. No more excuses, no more whining, just get going. I even gave you the Time-Savers chapter, so you no longer can use that as an excuse. But as I mentioned in my dedication to all of you right up front, this path is not for those who *need* it; but for those who *want* it. Want it enough to make self, health and sanity a priority.

If you choose *not* to follow this simpler path, I encourage you to take the "necessary" drugs recommended by your physician, have surgery as needed and enjoy life to the fullest for as long as you're on the planet. Either way, the choice is yours. And for the record, I believe either path can be "correct." Though I have seen hundreds of clients turn their health around with the methods I've suggested in this book, I'd be a fool to assure you with 100 percent certainty that they will work for you. That depends on you—and a hundred other factors that my crystal ball is keeping a secret. But keep in mind that doing nothing is a choice, too.

If you *do* choose to follow this path with the "merry band," to quote an awesome yoga teacher, John Friend, there are two things that will make it easier to continue making wise choices each and every day: celebrating the positive and making it fun.

Start celebrating each and every positive choice you make by writing them down daily. You can use your day planner to catch them moment by moment, or use a journal to record your healthy choices in the evening before bed right along with the blessings you experienced that day. It's true; what you focus on expands. So focus on the positive.

Secondly, make this is as fun as possible. Hey, isn't it fun to find out that quality fats are good for you, often decrease your sweet cravings and help you keep your weight balanced? And with the myriad of exercise choices available to you, surely there are two or three or twenty which are fun for you. You can find joy and beauty in a simple walk, whether it's cruising city streets, strolling on the beach or hiking in the woods.

And now, I'd like to share with you the wise words of a brand-new-to-me teacher, Betsy Downing. I am currently participating in the Anusara Yoga Gathering in Estes Park, Colorado where I met Betsy in a two-hour class devoted to handstands. I did them freely and joyfully in the grass as a kid, but now am learning them from a different perspective. It took me a few years to be able to kick up into a handstand against the wall, and Betsy helped me take this yoga pose to a new level yesterday.

For the first time, after 12 or 13 years of yoga practice, I was able to "push up" into a handstand from a wide-legged stance with just a tiny bit of assistance. Wow, what a way to celebrate my 50th birthday that's just around the corner! But that wasn't why Spirit/God/The Goddess had me sign up for that class. The real lesson came during Betsy's introduction.

I was a few minutes late to the class due to a potentially stressful lodging situation that took some time for me to work out. Thankfully, I had "only" felt stressed about it for 10 minutes or so before accepting the situation as is, and asking myself, "What are my choices now?" But I was still carrying a bit of that negative energy with me when I walked into the classroom. I try diligently to be on time to yoga classes, and especially at a large gathering, it feels even more important to be respectful of other participants and the instructor by being prompt. However, I was doing pretty well at accepting this aspect of life on life's terms when I walked in the door.

As I moved to the back of the room where there was still a little space for me, Betsy was talking about anger and frustration. She said that whenever we allow ourselves to feel them, we are removed from who we really are. As a recovering workaholic, recovering perfectionist and "fast twitch" kind of person, I knew she was talking to me. I smiled as I rolled out my mat, found my seat and listened with devoted attention. Hearing that reminder was why I was in class; pressing up into a handstand was just my treat for showing up.

Keep showing up, and stay tuned. I'm just getting started with uncovering who I really am. My next project is a yoga DVD with a booklet to keep it simple, and then … who knows? I'll keep showing up to find out.

As I close this, we are having a national election in just a few weeks. I hope you exercised your privilege to vote and I beg you to get out and vote every time that opportunity arrives. And when you do exercise your freedom to help choose our leaders, I encourage you to remember the words from my Christmas Carol hero, Tiny Tim.

God bless us, every one.

Appendix A

Multi-Drug Resistant Bacteria and Viruses

After a client of mine received an e-newsletter from our office about the bacteria and viruses which will not respond to any antibiotics or antivirals, she told me about an article in *Discover* magazine on this topic. When I searched for more information online, I was stunned by the results. Entering "killer bacteria" into their search engine revealed 46 articles on the subject, some going back to the early 1990's. When I typed in "killer virus," an additional 48 articles popped up, confirming my concern about this trend which began in the 1950's and is on the rise.

From a big picture point-of-view, these drug-resistant bacteria and viruses are a potential solution for overpopulation and our culture's apparent inclination to destroy our home—planet Earth. Bacteria have been around much longer than human beings and have killed large numbers of people on several occasions. Most recently, the influenza epidemic of 1918-1919 killed 675,000 Americans—more than the number of Americans killed in combat during World War I, World War II, Korea, and Vietnam *combined* (423,000). For more information, see *haverford.edu/biology/edwards/disease/viral_essays/redican-virus*. If you'd like to avoid being one of the humans these bacteria and viruses kill in their effort to resolve some of the world's problems, read on.

Protect Yourself Against MDR (Multiple Drug Resistance)

What the heck is MDR? You may have heard this referred to as MRSA (Multiple Resistance to Staphylococcus Aureus), which is similar to the bacteria that killed my friend, Debrah Rafel Osborn—a healthy and vibrant 48-year-old mother of twin babies—on Feburary 29, 2008. If you haven't seen articles in the news yet on these killer bacteria and viruses, you will soon.

First, let's explore the causes. Though antibiotics are life-saving in some situations, they have been overused to the point of killing many healthy bacteria that we need in order to live. This loss of beneficial bacteria lowers our immune response, making us more susceptible to any pathogen coming our way. Another reason these bacteria are becoming stronger is our recent love-affair with antibacterial products. The .01 percent survivors of anti-bacterial soaps, instant cleansers, and the like are mutating—it's like the human equivalent of weight-lifting and eating super foods. As of late summer, 2008, no antibiotic or antiviral drug was able to touch the very few bacteria that just won't die. Let's face it, folks; bacteria will win in the long term. They've been around a lot longer and are smarter, from an evolutionary point of view, than humans. But guess what type of remedies can save the day?

Yes, it's those simple plants that are often ignored as being ineffectual since they are usually taken in ineffective doses and/or forms. A few weeks after my friend, Debrah, died from one of these drug-resistant bacteria, I had the honor of being a student of David Winston's again—this time via the teleseminar, *Treatment of Bacterial MDR with Botanical Therapies* (See Bibliography). Here is some of what I learned:

◆ Medical causes of MDR include inappropriate use of antibiotics (often prescribed for *viral* infections), prophylactic use of antibiotics "just in case," and inadequate hygiene in medical settings.

◆ Environmental causes include amalgam fillings, exposure to pesticides, and pharmaceutical medications.

◆ Agricultural causes include widespread use of antibiotics in factory farming, use of antibiotics to enhance animal growth and many chemical sprays.

◆ Those with heightened risk include transplant patients, people with IV ports and those with any disease which suppresses the immune system. And of course, having any surgical procedure in any hospital or clinic.

Susan's Simple Tip

In 2005, 85 percent of these infections were associated with healthcare, but get this…14 percent were picked up in places like locker rooms and manicure spas. Before you get paranoid, let's have some good news: many antimicrobial herbs inhibit or kill MRSA when nothing else works! These include catnip, elecampane root, eucalyptus leaf, rosemary, garlic and osha root. Even more amazing are the herbs which *enhance* antibiotic activity: barberry root and leaf, bugleweed, eleutherococcus bark (aka Siberian ginseng), hops and a very favorite of mine, turmeric.

Do the following to protect yourself and others:

- ◆ Quit buying antibacterial products; regular soap and hot water is plenty effective, and won't kill the "good bacteria."
- ◆ Strengthen your immune response with regular exercise, garlic, cod liver oil, plenty of sleep, and a wholesome, healthy diet. Your immune system is the first line of defense.
- ◆ If manicures are a given for you, do your own and use the money you save for quality food— or a week on the beach.
- ◆ Wear flip-flops in the locker room and in community showers; wash your hands regularly when in public places.
- ◆ Minimize sugar and wheat in your diet and your pantry.

Appendix B

Digestion Basics

Digestion problems plague many individuals, usually due to lack of activity, poor food choices and the overuse of antibiotics. When a client does not respond to "tried and true" herbal remedies, I know we need to work on the gut. In fact, I usually include a digestive aid like ginger or cinnamon to most customized formulas right from the start. These carminative herbs, among many others, act as a "gut tonic" in addition to relieving gas and dispersing the rest of an herbal formula to the cells which need their help.

When the human body is unable to absorb nutrients from food and/or healing herbs, it usually indicates compromised digestion. Some of these gastrointestinal issues pop up during menopause since estrogen is a gastrointestinal stimulant; less estrogen can contribute indirectly to both gas and constipation. Bowel problems are the end result of an unhappy digestive system and important to regulate—without chronic use of laxatives, herbal or synthetic.

As always, I vow to keep this simple. Start with the most basic, and often free, changes to encourage better digestion. Follow the suggestions in each step for a week or two, adding the suggestions in subsequent steps if needed.

Step One

Give thanks for your food before you eat, acknowledging the plants and animals that nourish you, as well as all the people involved in bringing food to your table. Saying it out loud is best; inner thanks is fine when in a restaurant.

Susan's Simple Tip—
The Acid/Alkaline Conundrum:

I'm often asked about the acid/alkaline balance diet fad. I have not seen any solid research connecting the pH of saliva and urine to actual blood pH. Also, the statement often made that acidity helps microbes grow, does not square with the research showing that acidity in the stomach and on the skin kills germs. One thing I do know is that adequate protein, which I recommend at each meal, is very important in maintaining this balance.

Maintenance of proper pH in various parts of the body is a complex process involving many feedback loops and a variety of nutrients. Any time you test your pH, which is easy to do, the results are dependant on what you've had to eat and drink for the past few hours and days, plus many other factors. If I had to constantly check my pH to decide what to eat, I wouldn't get much done and besides—that would take all the fun out of eating! Follow this link to research the issue further: *WestonAPrice.org/letters/L2003sp*.

◆ Eat something every three to four hours to keep your blood sugar levels even and prevent you from gorging on junk food when you get too hungry.

◆ Eat at regular times and go to the bathroom at regular times—even if you don't feel the urge. You can read a tip from this book while waiting for your bowels to move. Give them at least five minutes.

◆ Drink hot water with fresh lemon at every meal and chew your food 20 to 30 times before swallowing. This tip alone usually makes a big difference, according to Deepak Chopra, M.D, and I concur. One-third of the digestive process takes place in your mouth, thanks to chewing and your saliva.

◆ Given our love affair with eating a low-fat diet, many people have constipation as a result of limiting high-quality, nutrient-dense fats such as coconut oil, animal fats, plain and whole yogurt, raw and whole milk. Try consuming raw foods like pineapples, bananas, papaya and fermented foods for digestive enzymes instead of doling out cash for yet another supplement. Check out these links for more information: *WestonAPrice.org/knowyourfats/fat_absorption* and *realmilk.com/enzyme.*

◆ If you have chronic constipation, heat a cup of hot water (or herbal tea) first thing in the morning, and take it back to bed. Sip it slowly while thinking about all your blessings. Then lie on your back and bend your knees with your feet flat on the bed; place your palms on your belly and breathe deeply. Gently begin to rub your belly in spirals: up on the right, across the middle, and down on the left. When you feel the movement gathering momentum, sit up slowly and head for the bathroom. Be patient.

◆ Any rhythmical exercise, especially walking, relieves digestive gas and encourages regular bowel movements—yet another reason to move.

◆ Plain, whole yogurt often helps with bloating and digestive gas—sometimes even a tiny mouthful will bring instant relief.

Step Two

◆ Drink a small glass of water with one teaspoon of raw apple cider vinegar added prior to each meal. In addition to enhancing digestion, this has been shown to help release extra weight over time— even without changes in diet or exercise.

◆ Chew or suck on fennel seeds whenever you feel some digestive discomfort—or when you need something to tide you over to your next meal.

◆ Processed flours, sugar and alcohol are often to blame for heartburn—especially when you're stressed. Remove these from your diet for a week or two; I predict you'll not only improve digestion, but release extra weight, too.

◆ Those same processed flours, along with too much grain-fed meat, slow the digestive tract and contribute to constipation. Whole grain products, well-cooked beans, wild meats, grass-fed beef and cooked greens speed it up.

◆ Are you taking iron supplements? Constipation and digestive distress are common side effects. Instead of expensive supplements, enjoy a spoonful of blackstrap molasses with 10-25 drops of yellow dock root tincture in a glass of warm water to increase iron and improve elimination. Yellow dock root tincture is also very helpful to menopausal women with digestive distress and highly recommended for women whose menses are getting heavier.

◆ Dandelion is the perfect ally for a happy digestive system and strong liver. It relieves indigestion, constipation, gas, even gallstone pain. Eat the omega-3-rich leaves in salads or take 10 to 20 drops of the tincture with meals. The tincture of the root is more helpful with constipation; the leaves are a natural diuretic.

◆ It's best for menopausal women to avoid the use of bran as a laxative since it interferes with calcium absorption. Instead, enjoy prunes, prune juice or figs.

◆ If constipation occurs due to fewer moistening, lubricating cells in the colon, slippery foods such as seaweed, flax seeds, and psyllium seeds (not the husk) are often helpful. Adding a teaspoon of any, or better yet, all of them to a cup of rolled oats and cooking until thick in three cups of water is a tasty way to consume a remedy.

◆ Acidophilus capsules are often helpful when dealing with chronic constipation or severe diarrhea. They help restore the healthy bacteria in the colon which is destroyed by antibiotics. But whole, plain yogurt is less expensive with a similar effect.

Step Three

◆ Add more liquids and soft foods to your diet to help relieve constipation. Examples include applesauce, yogurt, nourishing soups and herbal infusions. Drink three to four quarts of water and herbal teas throughout the day. Nettle tea (#58) rarely fails to assist with constipation.

◆ Ginger tea with raw honey is a soothing and warming drink when your tummy is upset. Try the fresh root grated and steeped in boiling water, or put a tablespoon of the powdered ginger from your spice cupboard in a cup of hot water and enjoy.

◆ Crushed hemp seed (Cannabis sativa) tea—rich in essential fatty acids—is a specific against menopausal constipation, according to Susun Weed. If you haven't found her resourceful web site yet, I encourage you to go to: *susunweed.com*. Her books are fabulous.

◆ Senna is a common ingredient in many of the popular detoxification products. Along with other herbal laxatives like the aloes and rhubarb root, it is addictive and destructive to normal peristalsis. I do not carry these in my dispensary and caution you to avoid them. I will occasionally use some cascara sagrada bark, an herbal laxative which is a little gentler, to help promote regular bowel movements. This is rarely needed if you follow the advice above.

Step Four

◆ Enemas and colonics are last-resort techniques. They do not promote health and may strip the gut of important microflora, an important part of your immune system. If you're considering colonics, be sure the practitioner adds the healthy bacteria back to the bowel. Regular use of enemas is highly habit-forming. Avoid both of these last-ditch options if at all possible. The only time I've had an enema is when I was nine and a half months pregnant at 178 pounds, and had not had a bowel movement in 10 days. God bless my mother for her help that day; it seemed to bring on labor, too!

Appendix C

Big Pharm's
Dirty Little Secret

What the Pharmaceutical Companies Don't Want You to Know

Most of us have never heard about an important number called NNT which stands for Number Needed to Treat. NNT answers the question, "How many people have to take a particular drug to avoid one incidence of a medical issue (such as a heart attack, or recurrence of cancer)?" For example, if a drug had an NNT of 50 for heart attacks, that means 50 people have to take the drug in order to prevent one heart attack. Looking at it another way, for every individual person who derives benefits from a drug, 49 will suffer the side effects with zero benefit.

First developed in 1988, NNT was intended to help you make a decision about whether or not to take a drug. Using the above example, for every 50 people who take a drug, perhaps one heart attack will be prevented, and the other 49 people will receive no benefit, puts things into perspective—a perspective the drug companies don't want you to see. That's why I'll bet you've never heard about this, right?

One of the most blatant examples of how drug companies have hidden NNT for their own self-serving purposes lies with cholesterol-lowering drugs. These drugs, which can cause side effects like liver damage, muscle weakness, cognitive impairment and many, many others, are touted as miracle pills that can slash your risk of a heart attack by more than one-third. *Business Week* did a story on this very topic, January 17, 2008, and they found the REAL numbers right on Pfizer's own newspaper ad for the cholesterol-lowering drug, Lipitor. Upon first glance, the ad boasts that Lipitor reduces heart attacks by 36 percent. However, there is an asterisk. And when you follow the asterisk, you find the following in much smaller type:

> "That means in a large clinical study, 3% of patients taking a sugar pill or placebo had a heart attack compared to 2% of patients taking Lipitor."

What *this* means is that for every 100 people who took the drug over 3.3 years, three people on placebos, and two people on Lipitor, had heart attacks. *That* means that taking Lipitor resulted in just one fewer heart attack per 100 people. So 100 people have to take Lipitor for more than three years to prevent one heart attack—and the other 99 people? They've just dished out thousands of dollars and increased their risk of negative side effects for nothing. Not to mention that this study was funded by the industry, which means their results may already be skewed, and the actual benefit may be even LESS than what they found.

In the *Business Week* article, Dr. Nortin M. Hadler, professor of medicine at the University of North Carolina at Chapel Hill, states, "Anything over an NNT of 50 is worse than a lottery ticket; there may be no winners." The NNT for some cholesterol-lowering drugs has been figured at 250 and up—even after taking those side-effect-laden drugs for five years!

Dr. Jerome R. Hoffman, professor of clinical medicine at the University of California in Los Angeles, asked *Business Week*, "What if you put 250 people in a room and told them they would each pay $1,000 a year for a drug they would have to take every day, that many would get diarrhea and muscle pain, and that 249 would have no benefit? And that they could do just as well by exercising? How many would take that?"

The answer, of course, is few to none. No wonder you have probably never heard of NNT before. Anytime you hear about how great a drug is, be suspicious. You wouldn't buy a car without finding out the real bottom line, right? Don't blindly accept the numbers that the drug companies peddle either.

One thing you can do is ask your doctor or pharmacist to tell you the NNT for any prescription you're currently taking, or considering. Even better, assume that most drugs offer little benefit and only take them as an absolute last option. Using the ever-popular statins as an example, **you could exercise regularly and take hawthorn tincture to protect your heart without all the side effects**. And empirically speaking, the NNT would be close to one. *You* have the power to take control of your health—and thrive—without pharmaceutical drugs. "Big Pharm" wants you to believe otherwise, but you know better. For more information on NNT, check out *mercola.com*.

Appendix D

My Favorite Foods

I let this book sit for at least a year after losing my original literary agent, Britt Tippins, when she had to unexpectedly move back to Europe for family reasons. Though I was frustrated and discouraged, I now know this was a blessing in many ways. One of the improvements I've made to the manuscript is this section. It may be seen as free advertising for certain products and I want you to know that is not my intention; I receive zero remuneration from the companies that produce the products listed in this Appendix, or any I've recommended. Actually— now that I'm thinking about it—there is one caveat to that statement. I do carry Standard Process products in my dispensary for the few clients who don't respond to better nutrition, exercise and herbs.

I know from personal experience how challenging it can be to find tasty and nutritious alternatives for the foods we've learned to enjoy. If you're intrigued by the short list you see below, go to the following website to learn how you can join "The Nutrition Information Army": *WestonAPrice.org/membership/infoarmy*.

When you become a member of this helpful non-profit organization, you can purchase an annually-updated Shopping Guide with lots more brand names for only a dollar. It's small enough to put in your purse or the glove compartment in your car.

Crackers—Ak-Mak, with only five wholesome ingredients, all of which I can pronounce, is the only whole-wheat cracker I've discovered that actually *tastes* good. However, now that I rarely eat wheat, I have discovered Mary's Gone Crackers, a tasty, non-wheat alternative.

Cold Cereal—none.

Yogurt—Brown Cow is the one in my area I prefer, but any quality organic, whole milk (NOT low-fat!) plain yogurt is a good choice. Add your own fruit or make a delicious smoothie with berries and any fruit in season. Yogurt made from raw milk is even better, but not always available.

Appetite "Suppressant"—fennel seeds not only help you curb your appetite at 5:00 P.M. when you're making dinner after a long and active day, but also promotes digestion.

Chocolate—the good stuff from Belgium uses only cocoa as its fat source. Godiva is my personal favorite; a little dab'll do ya.

Milk—I rarely drink milk—except with warm, whole-grain, chocolate chip cookies which are a very rare treat. Look for a raw dairy close to you, especially if you have milk-drinking children. Check out *realmilk.com* for more information.

Beef—no brand really, but whatever you can get that's been raised locally without antibiotics and hormones, and preferably slaughtered with respect. Grass-fed is best.

Chicken—Again no actual brand, raised without all the nasties and allowed to roam free. Support your local farms and ranches.

Fish—Salmon marinated in a little teriyaki sauce for a few minutes before grilling five minutes a side. This delicious and good-for-us fish has a healthy amount of omega-3's which are generally lacking in our diets (flax meal is good, too). There is a little sugar in teriyaki, but it's worth it to eat more fish—or some.

Potatoes—Yukon Gold since their lower in starch and delicious; they require less liquid for mashing than other potatoes.

Fresh Herb—One favorite? Of course, there's not just one; I'll list several starting with rosemary. She's the only one I can get to grow relatively well indoors; add rosemary's "remembrance" to soups, sauces, or sautéed anything to help prevent dementia and heart disease. Other favorites include: cilantro (delicious and great at helping prevent cancer); basil (what can I say—I was married to an Italian); and sage, since she mitigates hot flashes. If I were to include my favorite medicinal herbs we can enjoy in our food, there would be over a hundred actual favorites. Mother Nature has blessed us so. Choose the culinary herbs *you* are most drawn to, either by smell or flavor.

My Virtually Never Food List

Hydrogenated Oil—Also known as trans fatty acids (TFA's), this stuff is legal poison and only good for the food industry's bottom line. It's time to tell the truth about these legal poisons, and they're everywhere. Just try to find boxed "food" items at the supermarket without hydrogenated oil (any type of oil including the much-used soybean oil is nasty stuff when hydrogenated, and is a proven contributor to cancer). Any type of "vegetable" oil is actually just a tiny step less of a poison than hydrogenated oils. See *WestonAPrice.org* for details.

Fast Food—With a couple of exceptions, I do not eat fast food anymore. If I think it may be my only option on a busy day, I will take fruit, seeds or nuts with me plus a quart-size glass or stainless steel bottle of water wherever I'm going—empty if flying. This is especially true when I go on holiday; I'll take more food with me when I'm traveling because I know how tempting the burger joints can be. Exceptions: we have a local burrito place and also an Asian food restaurant that are sort of like fast food but made with wholesome and, overall, nutritious ingredients. I find that locally-owned places usually have better quality ingredients than chains. Ask them; and do your own research by asking locally-owned restaurants for ingredient lists.

Fried Food—Especially when eating at a restaurant that uses crappy (that's a scientific term) oil for deep frying. Start asking about the type of oil used in restaurants and you'll learn find that about 90 percent will respond with "vegetable oil" or worse yet, "fry oil." Again, this is code for poison. That's hydrogenated oil in a weak disguise. There are usually other options. If you focus on enjoying a quality protein, without extra sauces and with vegetables, you'll be miles ahead of the average American.

Appendix E

The Quick Six

After a decade plus in practice, I am realistic. Regardless of good intentions, if you can't keep healing simple, it's not going to happen. Even if you don't read all of *Take Back Your Body*, I want you to have some golden nuggets to help you lead a healthier—and simpler—life. The Quick Six offers short reminders to keep you on the path of personal responsibility for your health—without breaking the bank or eating up too much time. Commit to include at least one thing daily on this list of health reminders.

Number One—Rest

◆ If at all possible, get to bed by 10:00 P.M. and up by 6:00 A.M.. If you are in bed at 10:00 and wake up at 5:00 or 5:30 without an alarm, your body is telling you that you're getting the amount of sleep you need. Waking up without an alarm is infinitely better.

◆ Take short naps whenever you're feeling sluggish during the day—10 minutes can do wonders for your afternoon energy level.

◆ Sit and do nothing for five minutes a day— don't even meditate. Just gaze out the window or watch birds at a feeder. And breathe.

Joan had been a night owl for years, but when menopausal symptoms hit, she would wake up early without being able to go back to sleep. She was exhausted and cranky. Simply by adjusting her sleep schedule by going to bed earlier, she was able to get the rest needed for this important transition.

Number Two—Eat Well

◆ Consume five to seven fruits and veggies a day (a bit heavier on the veggies). No, McDonald's French fries do not count as a vegetable. But I admit they used to taste good before I found out what was in them by reading *Fast Food Nation*.

◆ Drink water—two quarts a day if you're averaged-sized and healthy; three to four quarts a day if you have health problems or you weigh more than 150 pounds. Chlorine-free and fluoride-free is best, but don't get too hung up on the details. Herbal teas count toward the total.

◆ Choose your vices wisely. For most Americans, it's unrealistic to expect total elimination. But do your best to limit the following: hydrogenated oils of all kinds, vegetable oils (don't worry; olives are a fruit and olive oil is a very healthy choice), white/processed flours, refined sugars of all kinds, soda, deep-fat fried foods, and any added chemicals including "natural flavors." Check all your labels carefully and ask questions of any restaurant. If you minimize these poisons, you'll feel no guilt with a beer or glass of wine or piece of good chocolate daily. When you make good choices 85 percent of the time, the other 15 percent is guilt-free and fun.

Marilyn came to see me about anxiety and panic attacks. Increasing her consumption of quality fats, along with eating something four to five times each day brought her back to calm.

Number Three—Move Your Body

- ◆ Shoot for this daily—to insure you get in some form of exercise at least four to five times a week. If you're sedentary now, start with a five minute walk. If you're already exercising two or three times a week, get outside for a 5 minute walk on the other days. Every day.
- ◆ For those who blanch at the thought of exercise, consider a gentle, beginner's yoga class or DVD for a multitude of benefits.
- ◆ Dancing counts—make it fun and mix up the activities.

Even without making dietary changes, Jim was able to start releasing extra weight just by walking for 20 minutes four or five times each week.

Number Four—Create Quiet Time

- ◆ I know, I know—you don't have time. My belief is that we all have time for the things that are important to us, but if you're convinced you don't even have five minutes a day to sit quietly, at least turn off the radio in your car and count the number of breaths it takes for you to drive to the market, work or your kids' school.
- ◆ Keep it simple. If the word "meditation" makes you break out into hives, just gaze out the window, observing the birds at a feeder or the leaves rustling in the breeze. Each time a distracting thought comes up, gently release it

and focus on your breath. Inhale and exhale through the nose, using a one-word mantra, such as "Peace" or "Relax." Be present.

Joanna, who is a true Type-A person, learned that she increased her productivity during the day when she carved out 15 minutes each morning for quiet time.

Number Five—Be Creative

◆ If you need support or encouragement to jump-start your creative side, consider joining a group that knits, quilts, reviews and discusses books, or looks for good stock-market buys. Consider reading *The Artists' Way* by Julia Cameron. It's an excellent resource—and not just for artists.

◆ No time for anything extra? Sing to the music in your car—regardless of how your voice sounds!

The clients I work with who are able to incorporate something creative into their daily lives respond faster and better to herbs and lifestyle changes than those who don't. Doodling while on the phone, writing, singing, dancing, painting, drawing, creative problem-solving—all count.

Number Six—Love Yourself and Others

◆ You can label this the "touchy-feely" part if you like—as long as you do it. If you're constantly beating up on yourself, all the healthy tips and smoothie recipes won't necessarily make a healthier you. Explore counseling if you need it

by asking for referrals or calling your local
mental health center.

◆ Whenever I'm stressed, I remind myself of my
top two priorities: serenity and compassion (for
myself and for others). My shoulders drop, I
breathe more deeply and usually remember
what's truly important in this life.

◆ One of the best ways to love yourself is to ask for
help when you need it. Many of us still function
with the Wild West mentality of being tough,
strong and independent—often to our own
detriment. We are blessed to have a multitude of
resources; use them!

I work with a lot of menopausal women who struggle to
put themselves first. Nancy, a mother of four teenagers,
shared with me that the only way she could carve out
quiet time was to remind herself that she is a better
mother when she's rested, well-fed and moving her body
regularly. She's also a better role model for her children
when practicing self care.

Ready for more? Scan the Table of Contents for the
tips of greatest interest to you. They are filled with
the how-to's of simple and healthy living that puts *you*
back in charge of your body.

Ginger Tea Baths—
The Overnight Cure
for the Common Cold

This "cure" for the common cold works every time, in my experience—if you do it correctly and do it soon enough. And I will say that your chances of it being effective go up if you are already taking care of yourself by eating whole foods and moving your body regularly.

Step One: Follow these instructions *the very first night* you feel any cold symptom. For me, it will be either a slight headache or a scratchy little cough that seems inconsequential. Do not wait until the second night!

Step Two: Prepare yourself for going to bed immediately after your bath. Call, or preferably email, your boss or the person you have your first appointment with the following day and alert them to your need to either come in to work late, due to illness, or postpone your appointment until the following day. Take any regular evening supplements or herbs, scrub your face, apply moisturizer, floss and brush your teeth, kiss your kids and/or significant other good night, lock up the cat or dog to minimize any nighttime disturbance.

Step Three: Make a fresh and strong ginger tea by grating about one tablespoon of fresh ginger into a tea ball or directly into a small tea pot. Ginger can be kept in the freezer for this purpose. Add freshly-boiled water, and a touch of raw honey if desired. Take this to the bathtub with you and allow it to steep while you draw a bath as hot as you can stand. Add some dead sea salts or Epsom salts, if desired, to your bath; not a requirement. Turn down your bed, and have a warm bathrobe right next to the tub. Turn off all lights, if possible, and light a candle.

Step Four: Step into the bath and submerge yourself up to the chin. Relax and enjoy the sweating heat as you drink the ginger tea. Ginger is a diaphoretic; it will help you sweat out the bacteria or virus responsible for the cold or flu you barely feel. Both are very susceptible to heat so this is a great way to move either a bacteria or virus through your body quickly. You will seriously start to sweat. Enjoy it and visualize your immune cells gaining strength and handling the bacteria or virus which is being killed off by the heat. Relax in the bath, counting your blessings or your breaths—avoiding any thoughts of the coming day—until the bath starts to cool a little.

Step Five: Get out of the bath, towel off quickly, put on your warm robe and go to bed immediately. Sleep as long as you can; no alarm allowed! Yes, you will feel warm. Yes, you will likely be sweating. And yes, your cold or flu should be gone the next day.

Step Six: Use some common sense the following day: take your time preparing for work, allowing your SO to take over with kids, if at all possible; take one or two 10-minute naps—under your desk if necessary; consume no sugar or alcohol on this day.

Repeat, as necessary, and thank Ric Scalzo, Founder of Gaia Herbs, for this simple and amazing remedy.

Bibliography

Addis, Paul. *Food and Nutrition News* 62(2), 7-10,
    March/April 1990.

Angelou, Maya. *Wouldn't Take Nothing for My Journey Now.*
    New York: Random House, 1993.

Appleton, Nancy. *Heal Yourself with Natural Foods.* New York:
    Sterling Publishing Co., Inc., 1998.

_____ . *Lick the Sugar Habit.* New York: Avery, 1996.

Barton, Anna M. *The Natural Pharmacist.* New York: Prima
    Publishing, 1999.

Beattie, Melody. *The Language of Letting Go.* New York: Harper
    Collins Publishers, 1990.

Beck, Martha. *The Joy Diet.* New York: Crown Publishers, 2003.

Beinfield, H., and Korngold, E. *Between Heaven and Earth.*
    New York: Ballantine Books, 1991.

Bone, Kerry. *A Clinical Guide to Blending Liquid Herbs.* New
    York: Churchill Livingstone, 2003.

_____ . *Principles and Practice of Phytotherapy* (with Simon
    Mills). New York: Churchill Livingstone, 2000.

_____ . *The Essential Guide To Herbal Safety.* New York:
    Churchill Livingstone, 2005.

Borysenko, Joan. *Inner Peace for Busy People.* Carlsbad: Hay
    House, 2003.

_____ . *Menopause: Initiation Into Power.* Carlsbad: Hay
    House, 2003.

Breathnach, Sarah Ban. *Simple Abundance.* New York: Warner
    Books, 1995.

Breus, Michael. *Good Night.* New York: Dutton Adult/Penguin
    Publishing Group, 2006.

Brinker, Francis. *Herb Contraindications and Drug Interactions.*
    Sandy: Eclectic Medical Publications, 1998.

Brizendine, Louann. *The Female Brain.* New York: Broadway
    Books, 2006.

Campbell, Jeff. *Speed Cleaning.* New York: Dell, 1991.

Chopra, Deepak. *Ageless Body, Timeless Mind.* New York:
    Harmony Books, 1993.

_____ . *Peace is The Way*. New York: Orbis Books, 2000.

_____ . *Perfect Health*. New York: Harmony Books, 1991.

_____ . *The Book of Secrets*. New York: Three Rivers Press, 2005.

_____ . *The Seven Spiritual Laws of Success*. San Rafael: Amber Allen Publishing, 1994.

Cohen, Kenneth. *Honoring the Medicine*. New York: Ballantine Books, 2003.

Couch, Jean. *The Runner's Yoga Book: A Balanced Approach to Fitness*. Berkeley: Rodmell Press, 1990.

Dacyczyn, Amy. *The Tightwad Gazette*. New York: Villard Publishing, 1998.

Deglin, Judith H. and Vallerand, April H. *Davis' Drug Guide for Nurses*, 8th Edition. Philadelphia: F. A. Davis Company, 2003.

Dossey, Larry. *Healing Words*. New York: Harper Collins Publishers, 1993.

_____ . *Reinventing Medicine*. San Francisco: Harper, 1999.

Fallon, Sally. *Nourishing Traditions*. Warsaw: New Trends Publishing, Inc., 1999.

Ferris, Timothy. *Four Hour Work Week*. New York: Crown Publishing, 2007.

Frawley, David and Lad, Vasant. *The Yoga of Herbs*. Twin Lakes: Lotus Press, 1986.

Gittleman, Ann L. *Before the Change, Taking Charge of Your Perimenopause*. San Francisco: Harper, 1998.

Gladstar, Rosemary. *Rosemary Gladstar's Family Herbal*. North Adams: Storey Publishing, 2001.

_____ . *Herbal Healing for Men's Health*. North Adams: Storey Publishing, 1999.

_____ . *Herbal Healing for Women*. New York: Fireside Publishing, 1993.

Grieve, Mrs. M. *A Modern Herbal*. London: Dorset Press, 1994 (first published in 1931).

Hanh, Thich Nhat. *Anger*. New York: Riverhead Books, 2001.

Hay, Louise L. *Heal Your Body*. Carlsbad: Hay House Publishing, 1984.

Hoffman, David. *Medical Herbalism*. Rochester: Healing Arts Press, 2003.

Holmes, Peter. *Jade Remedies*. Boulder: Snow Lotus Press, 1996.

_____ . *The Energetics of Western Herbs*. Boulder: Snow Lotus Press, 1983.

Hudson, Tori. *Women's Encyclopedia of Natural Medicine*. Los Angeles: Keats Publishing, 1999.

_____ . *Women's Encyclopedia of Natural Medicine*. New York: McGraw Hill, 1999.

Ito, Dee. *Without Estrogen*. New York: Crown Publishers, 1994.

Jarvis, J.C. *Folk Medicine*. Robinsdale: Fawcett Publishing, 1995.

Judith, Anodea. *Wheels of Life: A Users Guide to the Chakra System*. New York: Llewellyn Worldwide, Ltd., 1999.

Kaptchuck, Ted K. *The Web That Has No Weaver: Understanding Chinese Medicine*. New York: Congdon & Weed, 1983.

King, John. *The American Dispensatory*. Ann Arbor: University of Michigan Library Publishing, 1887.

Kingsolver, Barbara. *Animal, Vegetable, Miracle*. New York: Harper Collins Publishers, 2007.

Kloss, Jethro. *Back to Eden*. Loma Linda: Back to Eden Publishing Company, 1939.

Kornfield, Jack. *A Path With Heart*. New York: Bantam Books, 1993.

Lee, John R. *What Your Doctor May Not Tell You About Menopause*. New York: Warner Books, Inc., 1996.

Lonsdorf, Nancy. *A Woman's Best Medicine*. New York: Tarcher and Putnam, 1993.

Lopez, A. *American Journal of Clinical Nutrition* 18:149-53, 1966.

Love, Susan. *Dr. Susan Love's Hormone Book*. New York: Three Rivers Press, 1998.

McQuade, Crawford, Amanda. *Herbal Remedies for Women*. New York: Prima Publishing, 1997.

McIntyre, Anne. *The Complete Woman's Herbal, A Manual of Healing Herbs and Nutrition for Personal Well-being and Family Care*. New York: Henry Holt and Company, Inc., 1994.

McTaggart, Lynne. *What Doctors Don't Tell You*. New York: Avon Books, 1998.

Murray, Michael and Pizzorno, Joseph. *Encyclopedia of Natural Medicine*. New York: Prima Publishing, 1995.

Myss, Caroline. *Anatomy of the Spirit*. New York: Harmony Books, 1996.

Northrup, Christiane. *Women's Bodies, Women's Wisdom*. New York: Bantam Books Publishing, 1996.

_____ . *The Wisdom of Menopause*. New York: Bantam Books Publishing, 2006.

Nostrand, Carol A. *Junk Food to Real Food*. New Canaan: Keats Publishing, 1994.

O'Connor, Dagmar. *How To Make Love To The Same Person for the Rest of Your Life and Still Love It*. New York: Bantam Books Doubleday Dell Publishing Group, 1985.

Orloff, Judith. *Guide to Intuitive Healing*. New York: Three Rivers Press, 2000.

Oz, Mehmet, and Roizen, Michael. *You: The Owners Manual*. New York: Harper Collins Publishing, 2005.

Physicians' Desk Reference, 2006 Edition. Williston: Thomas PDR, 2006.

Pitchford, Paul. *Healing with Whole Foods*. Berkeley: North Atlantic Books, 1993.

Sheehy, Gail. *Silent Passage*. New York: Pocket Books, 1993.

St. James, Elaine. *Simplify Your Life*. New York: Hyperion Publishing, 1994.

_____ . *The Simplicity Reader*. New York: Smithmark Publishers, 1998.

Steinem, Gloria. *Moving Beyond Words*. New York: Simon and Schuster, 1994.

Tierra, Michael and Tierra, Leslie. *Chinese Traditional Herbal Medicine*. Twin Lakes: Lotus Publishing, 1998.

_____ . *Treating Cancer with Herbs*. Twin Lakes: Lotus Press, 2003.

_____ . *Planetary Herbology*. Twin Lakes: Lotus Publishing, 1988.

_____ . *The Herbs of Life*. New York: Crossing Press, 1992.

Tolle, Eckhart. *A New Earth*. New York: Dutton Adult, 2005.

Weed, Susan. *Breast Cancer? Breast Health*. New York: Ash Tree Publishing, 1996.

_____ . *Healing Wise*, New York: Ash Tree Publishing, 1989.

_____ . *The New Menopausal Years*. New York: Ash Tree Publishing, 1992.

Weil, Andrew. *8 Weeks to Optimum Health*. New York: Alfred A. Knopf, 2000.

_____ . *Eating Well for Optimum Health*. New York: Alfred A. Knopf, 2000.

_____ . *Self Healing Newsletters*.

Weschler's, Tomi. *Taking Charge of Your Fertility*. New York: Harper Collins Publishers, 1995.

Williams, David. *Alternatives for the Health-Conscious Individual. The True New Miracles for Men*. West Virginia: Mountain Home Publishing, 2006.

Winn, Marie. *Unplugging the Plug-in Drug*. New York: Penguin Publishing, 1987.

Winston, David. *Treatment of Bacterial MDR with Botanical Therapies*. Ashland: Herbal Educational Services, 2008.

Yance, Donald R. Jr. *Herbal Medicine, Healing and Cancer*. Chicago: Keats Publishing, 1999.

Yudkin, J., et al. *Annals of Nutrition and Metabolism* 30(4), 261-66, 1986.

_____ . *Sugar: Chemical, Biological and Nutritional Aspects of Sucrose*. 1971, Hartford: Daniel Davey.

Yudkin, J. *The Lancet*, 11, 155-62, 1957.

Index

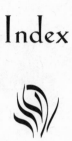

About the Author

Susan Mead was born in Lynn, Massachusetts, just outside of Boston, and raised in Scottsbluff, Nebraska. After graduating as a Cornhusker from the University of Nebraska with a B.S. degree in Business Administration, 1980, Susan emigrated to Fort Collins, Colorado, where she has spent most of her adult life.

After several jobs in marketing, sales and management in the 1980s, she started Team Techniques, an Organizational Development firm, where she used the Myers-Briggs Type Indicator and other teambuilding tools to help management and workers build bridges. But an internet start-up company convinced her to become their third employee as Director of Marketing, which she enjoyed until the venture capitalists dramatically changed the organization 16 months later.

After experiencing the business world for nearly 20 years, Susan's passion for helping others heal themselves became more personal when she walked into an herbal apothecary in Durango, CO, and instantly felt "at home." Looking for a saner way to contribute to our world than 60-hour work-weeks, Susan was simultaneously being tapped on the shoulder by the spirit of her great-grandmother, Sarah Fowler, who had signed on as a cook with the railroad as a way to respectably head West in the 1800s. When the railroad workers became ill or had an injury, Miss Fowler used her knowledge of simple plants to help the workers heal.

Though Susan had studied herbal remedies and nutrition for many years to enhance her own health, she now considered making her passion a profession which would honor her great-grandmother's knowledge. Juggling the demands of herbal medicine school with her full-time job was a challenge, but she sees the rewards for that commitment in the eyes of each individual who finds healing through simple and effective ways.

As *Take Back Your Body* goes to print in the fall of 2008, after nine years of gestation, Susan is clear that her background in business and public speaking helped guide her to her true purpose: writing and speaking about health care. In addition to these ongoing efforts, she continues to work with established clients—many of whom have been with her since 1996, when she established her practice. Susan also works part-time in Steamboat Springs as a volunteer for the Courtesy Ski Patrol.

Information on her dynamic speaking presentations, writing, yoga DVDs and her "tell-it-like-it-is" approach to moving from health care to self care can be found on her website at *SusanEMead.com*. And when you are there, sign up for her free electronic newsletter for a fresh perspective on health care issues in today's news.

Susan E. Mead, M.H.
Speaker, Writer, Master Herbalist and Yoga Instructor
www.SusanEMead.com

Notes

Notes

Notes

Notes